THE BECOMING BULLETPROOF PROJECT

Discovering the Hero Within

BY TIM ANDERSON

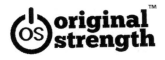

The Becoming Bulletproof Project:Discovering the Hero Within

by Tim Anderson

Copyright © 2019 Original Strength Systems, LLC

Published by OS Press

Edition ISBNs:
Paperback: 978-1-64184-077-4
ebook: 978-1-64184-078-1

First Edition 2019
Printed in the United States of America

Thank you to JETLAUNCH.net for editing and book design.

CONTENTS

DISCLAIMER!

You must get your physician's approval before beginning this exercise program.

These recommendations are not medical guidelines but are for educational purposes only. You must consult your physician prior to starting this program or if you have any medical condition or injury that is contraindicated to performing physical activity. This program is designed for healthy individuals eighteen years and older only.

See your physician before starting any exercise or nutrition program. If you are taking any medications, you must talk to your physician before starting any exercise program, including The Becoming Bulletproof Project. If you experience any lightheadedness, dizziness, or shortness of breath while exercising, stop the movement and consult a physician.

It is strongly recommended that you have a complete physical examination if you live a sedentary lifestyle, have high cholesterol, high blood pressure, diabetes, are overweight, or if you are over thirty years old. Please discuss all nutritional changes with your physician or a registered dietician. If your physician recommends that you not use The Becoming Bulletproof Project, please follow your doctor's orders.

All forms of exercise pose some inherent risks. The authors, editors, and publishers advise readers to take full responsibility for their own safety and know their limits. When using the exercises in this program, do not take risks beyond your level of experience, aptitude, training, and fitness. The exercises and dietary programs in this program are not intended as a substitute for any exercise routine, treatment, or dietary regimen prescribed by your physician.

TO THE BULLETPROOF

This book is dedicated to the bulletproof ones who have inspired me. With your courage, conviction, and gentleness you have shaped my life and opened my eyes to limitless possibilities; you've taught me how to fly.

Thank you, John Brookfield, Dan John, Freddie Mitchell, Trey Baker and Dad.

IN THE BEGINNING...

"*They can be a great people, Kal-El; they wish to be. They only lack the light to show the way. For this reason above all, their capacity for good, I have sent them you... my only son.*"
—Jor-El, Superman

I'm a little weird. All my life, I've wanted to be Superman. I'll admit, there was a brief stint of wanting to be Batman when I was four, but other than then, I've wanted to fly and be bulletproof. I didn't think that too weird when I was nine, but when I turned thirty, I started to wonder if it was "normal." I never seemed to outgrow that desire like others seemed to. As a full-grown adult, I still fantasize about saving the day, doing the right thing, and being impervious to injury.

Be honest. At some point in your life, you have wanted super-strength. You've wanted to pick up something really heavy like a cow or jump over something really big like a car. Or maybe you've actually wanted to rescue someone from a tragic situation. It's perfectly natural to want to be strong. It's natural because we are designed to be strong. In fact, the blueprint for superhuman strength lives inside of our nervous system. It's inside of us, waiting for us to tap into it. I believe that's where the natural desire comes from, it's calling on us, or asking us to let it out. We just don't recognize it as anything more than a childish thought or a weird daydream, so we dismiss it. But it is there, inside of us.

Fortunately for me this desire to be bulletproof never really left me alone. It was always there making itself known. In a *wild* way, this led to the discovery of a book called *Wild at Heart* by John Eldridge. In the book, Eldridge says that every man is born with the desire to be a hero, or the desire to "have what it takes." Phew, ok, I'm not that weird. It's completely natural for me to want to be Superman.

It's natural, but is it realistic?

Yes, I think so. And that's what this book is about. I do believe it is realistic for any of us to become the "super" hero we want to be. Maybe not actually fly — though more and more with technology that seems to be very doable — but perhaps we can all become bulletproof; able to overcome anything, able to be physically and mentally resilient, strong, and powerful, able to heal quickly, able to do the right thing because we can, able to save the day on any day. I believe we can all live this way, but I also believe we were all *made* to live this way.

You might be thinking, "Yep. He is a weirdo. I don't care what he believes." And that's cool, this book may not be for you. But if you are anyone who has ever wanted to be stronger than you are, or if you are anyone who has ever wanted or wondered if they "have what it takes," or if you are anyone who has ever wanted to be capable — physically able and willing — of doing the right thing to "save the day" then this book is for you.

The Becoming Bulletproof Project is about becoming who we were meant to be, about becoming who we are created to be. Becoming... Project... As these two words may suggest, it is an active process without a finish line. The more we become, the more we are able to reach for, and the more we are able to seek. And that's life. It has a starting point, and from there we are supposed to build and grow and become more than we were.

That may not be your take on life yet, and that's ok. You may be thinking, "Yes, there is a starting point. And we do become more, but then we peak. Then we decline. Then we break. Then we die..." I will agree with you that scenario seems to be prevalent and all around us. But I will encourage you to be open to the idea that just because things seem commonplace does not mean that is the way things are supposed to be.

Stay with me. I'm not saying we won't die. I'm saying that perhaps we were created to die with strength. Perhaps we were created to be able to "save the day" right up to the day we leave this world, whether that be in service to others or in a natural exit. I'm not the only one who thinks this way and there are examples of this happening throughout history. My friend Steve Holliner, a strength coach, even created a business based on this belief called "Die Mighty."

The point is, we were each created to become bulletproof. We were all meant to live a life of strength and vigor; able to live like warriors, heroes, saints, and servants. We were all made to "save the day," to make it better, whatever that may look like. And, we all have what it takes, if we choose to. If we choose to become...

This is important to note. We can all be superheroes. But Becoming Bulletproof is a choice.

We each have immeasurable potential and power within us. But the choice to let it out, the choice to use it, the choice to nurture it — that all takes energy, determination, willingness, and even surrender.

Sometimes the choice to become bulletproof is proactive. Sometimes the choice is reactive. Life is funny, it has a way of throwing events and situations at us that cause us to respond. Sometimes we don't know what we are capable of until we are faced with situations that demand we fall and yet something in us demands we rise.

Having said that, it is obvious that becoming bulletproof is much more than physical ability. It's much more than mental ability too. There are many variables that dance together to collectively influence the expression of our superhuman abilities.

Though we will focus more on the physical side of things, we will be taking a look at each of these: how we move, how we think, what we believe, how we learn, and the life that goes on around us — all of these influence our ability to overcome and withstand the effects of time throughout our lives here on earth.

In the following chapters I am going share with you what I've learned about becoming bulletproof and how I'm still going about it. I would like to draw your attention to the word *becoming* again. I am constantly in process. I am much further than where I once was, but I know I'm still learning how to fly...

Learning to Fly

Sometimes it takes being stupid to seek wisdom. Stupidity can cause a great deal of suffering but once a person gets tired of suffering they become open to different ways of thinking — at least this has been my own personal experience.

In my youth, I did some unintelligent things in the guise of "strength training" when it came to pursuing my desire to be Superman. Some of this I can attribute to "just not knowing any better," but even still, most of it was blind ignorance.

I was very steeped in the bodybuilding mentality of strength training. What I really mean is I benched a lot. Sets, reps, nausea, repeat. Every day. From the time I was 13 years old to the time I was 30 — I'll wager I didn't miss more than 10 days of "working out" in all of those years. It was a weird sickness. I think I somehow believed atoms would divide if I missed a day of training. If I traveled, the first line of business was to find a gym. I would actually leave my family for 2 or more hours every day while on vacation if it meant I could work out.

I was really stupid. There was no prize to be had, other than an ego check. I had a ravenous desire to be "strong" and it became my identity. If I didn't work out, if I missed one day, my self-esteem would tank. My misguided notion and quest to be strong motivated most all my decisions. I was lost...

As it won't surprise you, a sickness like the one I had can lead to other issues. I developed "itises." Tendonitis, swelling, pulled muscles — for years I ignored them or pushed through them. They were badges of honor. I didn't train around them, I didn't let them heal. I used ice, ibuprophen, and wraps. Until I couldn't. Eventually, and fortunately, my "itises" started interrupting my ability to train as well as my ability to do simple things like open a refrigerator door. My blind pursuit of strength had begun affecting my quality of life. The truth is, I was breaking myself. The deeper truth is, most of my life I had been living under a misguided, delusional and unconscious spell: I mislabeled my identity to be what I did instead of who I was. That, and I didn't understand the pull or the call that was inside of me fueling my devotion to never miss a day of training. Some of you reading this will understand what I just said, for those that don't, I'll talk about it later.

Anyway, the beautiful thing about pain is that it can often wake you up out of a deep sleep and I had been asleep for years. Pain led to frustration. Frustration led to despair. I was waking up and my reality was starting to suck — I wasn't Superman. I was broken. My thoughts were damaged, my body was damaged. It could have been much worse. I can't tell you I suffered from anything horrible other than the thoughts in my head. But it took these thoughts of brokenness to wake me up. This is where I began to learn how to fly.

I was awake to the point that I didn't want to hurt and I wanted to be able to do the things I wanted to do. So, I embarked on a journey of trying to heal myself. And I learned a lot. But the more I learned, the more frustrated I became because I just could not fix myself no matter what I had learned. I remember one night, I was very unsettled in my thoughts. I was feeling fragile, but at the same time I was holding onto a notion that I wasn't supposed to be fragile. So, I threw up a Hail Mary — I asked God a question: Would you show me how to train to become bulletproof?

That was nine years ago, as I am writing this today. What I've learned and what I've been able to do has been nothing short of miraculous. I can tell you without reservation, we were all meant to fly and we all have what it takes. It's inside each of us.

THE ORIGINAL BLUEPRINT

"The question is, which pill will you choose?"
— Morpheus, The Matrix

Superhuman strength and durability are actually programed or embedded inside of your nervous system. As an infant you were programed with a series of reflexes and movement patterns all intended to give you the strength and ability to be super-human. Along with these movements, even the very shape of your body was designed to give you amazing strength. If you consider the disproportionately oversized head of an infant and the ultimate mastery and control they eventually learn to balance it over their bodies with, you can start to see the human body is capable of fantastic feats. Don't get me wrong, there are certainly plenty of bumps and bruises along the way, but they are part of the process of gaining head control; head control demanded from the "righting reflex" that is programed inside of the infant.

The point is, we are all born with an original operating system or an original blueprint intended to connect our bodies and make us very hard to break. For three or more years we patiently worked our way through these programs, reflexes and patterns simply by learning how to move and position ourselves against gravity. But that was just the beginning, the birth of our superhuman strength. It was never meant to be the end of it.

Have you ever noticed how durable young children are? They can take horrible falls or terrible spills, and often shake it off and get back to playing, though sometimes after expressing their hurt or anger in tears. Kids seem to know how to express emotion and move on — that's part of being bulletproof as well. Anyway, children are fantastically resilient. Until they learn how to not move. Once a child learns how to sit all day long, all the wonderful work that happened during the first three years of their lives can begin to unravel. Instead of continuing to get stronger and more athletic, they stagnate or backslide in coordination. If this continues into adulthood, you end up with "fragile" adults; no strength, no energy, no endurance, no ability to cope with stress, no hope, no....

But that's not the way it should be, and deep down inside you know this. Does it make any sense for the most resilient years of our lives to be the first three? For those of you with an athletic background, does it make any sense that the first twenty years of our lives are the years we were strong and fast? Why would a human being have a lifespan of 80 to 120 years but only be strong and able for the first twenty? Why would our design allow "things to fall apart once you turn thirty" if we still had another 50 to 60 years of life left to live?

The original internal blueprint says that's not the design. Our developmental sequence says we are to be developed — throughout life. We don't erase our original blueprint as we age, it's still inside of us. Why then, are so many people broken? Why are backs, knees, and shoulders so fragile? Why are there so many people in rest homes, unable to take care of themselves? If we are all meant to be superhuman, WHERE are all the superhumans?

They are forgotten, abandoned, and locked away inside. They began to disappear once man forgot he was designed to move. The evidence of superhumans is everywhere in our history and our art, from times long forgotten. Where once we built pyramids with our hands, we can now build towers with cranes. Where once soldiers could march 18 to 25 miles per day and then conquer other countries, now many soldiers suffer injuries while taking physical fitness tests.

Times have changed. Technology, as great and fantastic as it is, has replaced the need for us to move as we are designed and able to move. So we bury our design, we forget how to move, and we become fragile. Add to that the new "normal", the commonplace issues of our day like obesity, diabetes, Alzheimer's, dementia, arthritis, heart disease and so on, and it becomes hard to remember something deeper within ourselves.

If all you see is the commonplace, if all you hear about is how the body falls apart as you age, you may start to believe these are the normal courses of life and that's just the way things are. No wonder superhero movies are so popular now. They are the number one revenue generating genre of the 2000s so far, with no end in sight. This is not an accident, it's a cry to be discovered. We all know there is something more; we all want to be something more. We can't help it — our blueprint wants to carry out its design. But we ignore it, or we fantasize it and create stories of heroes or flock to see stories of heroes. Why? Because Like attracts Like and Kind attracts Kind. We are drawn to what we are.

Remembering Our True Selves

What we are is a powerful moving masterpiece capable of fantastic feats of selfless heroism, endless creativity, and infinite expression. The truth is, we are much more than that, but how can you articulate the indescribable? The point is, inside your body is a program designed to be carried out so that you can live a life of true strength without limits. This program never leaves you, it's always in you, regardless if you haven't used it in twenty to fifty years. All you have to do for the program to take effect and begin restoring your true self is to engage in it.

This original blue print or program is actually designed to be carried out moment by moment, movement by movement throughout your entire life. I've written extensively about it in *Pressing RESET: Original Strength Reloaded.* You can learn more about it there. Here, I would like to talk about the essence of the blue print; The Three Pillars of Human Movement. These three pillars have been embedded in the developmental sequence of every child that has ever been born. They are the physical keys to becoming bulletproof and living a life of strength and health. Here they are:

1) Breathe properly with your diaphragm by keeping your tongue on the roof of your mouth and breathing through your nose.

2) Activate your vestibular system through controlling the movements of your head, including your eye movements and tongue movements.

3) Engage in your contra-lateral gait pattern, deliberately and reflexively using all four limbs to crawl, walk, or run.

These are the Pillars of Human Movement and they are essential to becoming bulletproof. If we engage in these three things regularly we will rediscover our strength and ability to move with ease and fluidity. We will also lower our risk of injuries and we can even recover from injuries faster. Though I've talked about how to Press RESET with these pillars of movement in other books, I want to take a deeper dive with them here through talking about the importance of the tongue.

The Rudder that Guides the Ship

The tongue is truly the most powerful muscle in the human body. It has power through influence to be more exact. You probably already know the tongue has the ability to save a life or start a war through words, but did you know the tongue influences how the body moves?

? = Fact check This

?? Holding your tongue where it belongs, or keeping
designed resting position, affects everything about he
body moves; from the posture in which you carry yourself to
the power you can produce through your muscles. The tongue
even influences the autonomic state of your nervous system,
whether you are in "fight or flight" mode or "rest and digest"
mode (it can influence whether or not you are stressed out).

The tongue is designed to rest against the roof of your mouth.
If you don't know where this resting place is, just swallow. Your
tongue will naturally go there. That is where it should spend the
majority of its time. That is where it carries the most positive
influence in your body.

Considering the natural resting position of the tongue, let's
look at the Three Pillars of Human Movement.

The Tongue and Breathing

? The tongue is neurologically connected to the diaphragm.[1] That
means they are closely involved and related to each other. To
see how this might be so, let's test it out.

Remove your tongue from the roof of your mouth and
rest it on the bottom of your mouth. Take a big inhalation in
through your nose, as big as you can. Now, place your tongue
on the roof of your mouth and take a big breath in through
your nose. Which breath was easier? Now fold your tongue in
half and press the bottom of your tongue against the roof of
your mouth. Take a big inhalation in through your nose, as big
as you can. Was that breath even easier?

How you hold your tongue affects how your diaphragm
works. Resting your tongue where it belongs optimizes your
diaphragms ability to function properly. This is so important
because the diaphragm is like the captain of all your spinal stabilizing muscles. If your diaphragm is getting optimal information
because your tongue is in the right place, then your pelvic floor
is also going to be getting optimal information, increasing its
likelihood of functioning properly. In other words, the tongue
is very influential in whether or not your inner core muscular

unit, your spinal stabilizers, are functioning properly — this is called reflexive strength.

What this means is if your tongue is where it belongs, you have a greater likelihood that your spinal stabilizers are functioning properly. This means your body will be free to move well and produce power. This also means your body will be less likely to be stiff or immobile, which means you'll be less likely to get injured from day to day activities.

I know this sounds nuts but holding your tongue where it is meant to be could be the beginning of rediscovering your physical strength and even restoring your body's health.

The Tongue and the Vestibular System

? The tongue is also neurologically connected to the vestibular system. In truth, EVERY muscle in your body is connected to your vestibular system. And the vestibular system is connected to every muscle. The relationship is quite chicken and egg, but the point is, the tongue provides more complete information to the brain via the vestibular system. Your vestibular system is the body's balance system and the body's information cross-roads system. All information generated and received by the body goes to the brain after traveling through the vestibular system. The brain takes that information and returns "instructions of response" back through the vestibular system out into the body. In other words, the brain tells the body what to do based off the information it receives from the vestibular system. A healthy vestibular system is CRUCIAL to living a life of health and strength. Without a healthy vestibular system, you cannot access your superpowers.

Again, the tongue provides more complete information to the brain through the vestibular system. If you were tracking with the information about the tongue and the diaphragm, then you might be able to see how the tongue provides information to the brain about the health of the spinal stabilizers too. Everything is connected to everything and it all matters. Where you hold your tongue greatly influences your vestibular system and provides it with optimal information, keeping the vestibular system healthy.

Remembering the second Pillar of Human Movement, how you hold your tongue, how you control your tongue is a part of controlling the movements of your head. If you have excellent head control, you more than likely have excellent balance, posture, and coordination. In fact, people who don't keep their tongue on the roof of their mouth tend to have poor posture; their head often protrudes out in front of their body and their back is often hyper-lordotic. Simply keeping the tongue on the roof of the mouth can help reverse this. But don't miss this, everything about you dances together. If your posture is good, your balance is good, your coordination is likely good, your mobility is good, and strength and power are good also. Every quality of movement influences every quality of movement. It's a beautiful dance...

To see how this might be so, let's test it out. Stand up and place your right palm on your right thigh. We are going to test your right shoulder's flexion range of motion and quality of motion. Open your mouth, hold your tongue on the bottom of your mouth, and raise your right arm up towards your right ear (keep your elbow locked and see how close your arm can get to your ear by raising it up from the front of your thigh). Notice how far your arm could travel towards your ear and how it felt. Now, close your mouth, place your tongue on the roof of your mouth where it belongs and raise your arm the same way. Which way felt better? With which way did you have more range of motion from your arm? Now, keeping your lips closed, fold your tongue in half and press the bottom of your tongue against the roof of your mouth and test the same movement again. Did it also feel different? Was your shoulder able to move further with more ease of movement? More than likely, you noticed a marked difference. But by placing your tongue on the roof of your mouth, your shoulder doesn't just move better, all of you moves better. In fact, a study conducted in 2013 demonstrated that tongue placement, specifically placing the tongue on the roof of the mouth, could improve power output of knee flexion by 30%.[2] Can you imagine being able to improve your power output by 30% simply by keeping your tongue on the roof of your mouth?

The Tongue and The Gait Pattern

If tongue placement affects how we breathe and how our spinal stabilizers function, and it also affects our posture and the quality of our movements, then it is easy to understand how tongue placement can affect and influence the gait pattern. How efficient we walk, how fluid we run, how fast we tire, how much power we produce with our stride — it is all influenced by where we keep our tongue. It matters. The tongue is "the rudder that guides the whole ship."

It is also easy to see how the Three Pillars of Human Movement are meant to be intertwined or woven together. They are a package deal. Done together, braided together, they keep us strong and resilient. They made us resilient the first three years of life and they are intended to develop us and strengthen us throughout our entire lives.

Here is the bottom line, and it's a deep line: If you can't control your tongue, you can't be bulletproof.

The tongue and the Three Pillars of Human Movement — this is your foundation, this is your design. This is the beginning of strength…

WHAT IS REAL STRENGTH?

"I can't lose you again! I can't. Not again. I'm not... strong enough."
— Mr. Incredible, The Incredibles

There are numerous definitions and opinions about what strength is and what it is not. Strength is something I've been trying to define for myself for the last several years. I think I've finally rested on what I believe strength to be: Strength is the ability to live life the way you want to live it; to be able to move, think, work, play, love and laugh throughout your entire life, regardless of your age. I will admit, my definition of strength is extremely hard to quantify. In fact, only one person is qualified to quantify it: YOU. Ultimately, you are the one who determines whether or not you are strong enough to live the way you want to live. No one else should be the judge of your own personal strength, no one else can live the life that you want to live. This can actually be quite a freeing thought if you have ever been around the "You have to deadlift 3-times your bodyweight to be considered 'strong'" group. That's a very narrowminded group, by the way.

Anyway, as evident from my definition of strength, it is more than a physical characteristic. To be sure, muscular strength plays a huge role in "strength", but so does mental strength. In fact, mental strength — the ability to endure, focus, withstand, and think — can ultimately trump physical strength. The mind can, does and will lead the body. The thoughts you hold in your head determine the course your body will end up taking. A strong mind can produce a very strong body and a weak mind will lead to a frail body. They are a package deal. One influences the other, though the mind has more "weight" behind it. When a person has a strong mind, they can effectively develop a strong body. Then they can pretty much engage in life to the level of their desire. **This is strength.**

In our quest to become bulletproof and unleash our inner super-powers, we will be looking at developing both mental and physical strength together.

The Strength of an Ox

Physical strength is a blessing. Having it enables us to do so many things that we take for granted like carrying in the groceries, climbing the stairs, getting up from the floor, playing tag with our kids and so on. In truth, physical strength leads to enjoying life.

It does at least, if it is not held in extremes. There are extremes to everything, even physical strength. One man can be strong enough to pick up 1000 pounds from the floor. Another man can be strong enough to run 100 kilometers without stopping (yes, that is an example of amazing mental strength too). These can both be areas of strength extremes.

For example, the man strong enough to pick up 1000 pounds may be completely winded after he climbs up one flight of stairs. He may even have to stop and catch his breath before he even reaches the top of one flight. That is a sign of great absolute strength, but not so great enduring strength (strength endurance). The other man who can run for 100 kilometers may lack the strength to deadlift his own bodyweight. This is an example of great strength endurance, but not so great absolute strength.

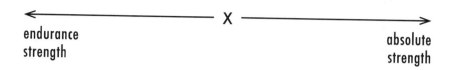

endurance
strength

absolute
strength

Imagine strength as a continuum line with the ends of the line being extreme strength endurance and extreme absolute strength. Ideally, we need to be somewhere in the middle. We want balance. When it comes to physical strength, we really don't need to live in the extremes. We need a good balance of strength. We don't have to live in the exact center of the line, but it is great if we are somewhere close to the middle.

Possessing both absolute strength *AND* strength endurance is a great place to live. That is the place that allows you to survive life's adventures and hardships. Having this balance, living somewhere in the middle of the strength continuum line, is what allows you to be an overcomer. To be prepared for all that life throws at you, you want to have both a high amount of absolute strength and a high amount of strength endurance. In other words, you want to have the strength of an ox.

An ox has a tremendous work capacity. Oxen can pull a tremendous load all day without tiring. An ox has muscle that won't quit. That is the type of muscle you want to have: Muscle that has the capacity to do large volumes of work and never tire. That is also the type of muscle that conventional strength and endurance training may not give you.

I have witnessed this first hand. Many moons ago, I was a firefighter. In my time as a firefighter, I learned one very important life-saving piece of knowledge: I wanted to be partnered up with a farm boy. The farm boys never tired out in a house fire. I witnessed very powerful, muscular men become completely exhausted in 5 minutes, but the farm boys could last for hours and never tire. If you have to go into a dangerous situation that requires a lot of physical effort you want two things:

1. You want to have the physical ability to endure whatever the situation throws at you.

2. You want the guy beside you to also have the physical ability to endure whatever the situation throws at him.

You don't want to have to think that your partner can't "take the heat", or that he is going to get so wiped out physically that he is in danger or a danger to you. On the flip side of that, should something happen to you, you want to know that your partner is capable of getting you to safety.

Farm boys make great firefighters because they don't typically train in the conventional strength training world. They just work. They work from sun up to sun down. They carry things, move things, feed things and milk things. They may count cows, but they don't count reps. They simply work. Their bodies are strong, and their minds are strong because they are accustomed to working long hours in order to complete the tasks of the day. They don't set aside an hour to strength train, but instead may set aside an hour to rest. This type of work load not only strengthens the body, but it also conditions the mind.

Traditional strength training, whether it is in the realm of power-lifting, bodybuilding, or the sport of weight lifting, does not prepare you for the rigors of life. Don't misunderstand, traditional strength training has its place, but it will not necessarily give you the strength you need to succeed in life. It will not give you the strength of an ox, or a farm boy. It may actually make your body "weaker" because it can actually weaken your mental fortitude.

Now you may be wondering, "*How can traditional, physical strength training weaken your mental strength?*" Take a deep breath as you read this: *Always* allowing rest breaks, *always* stopping a task when things get difficult, always changing a task every 30 seconds, are all ways that can weaken your mental resolve because you are simply *always* telling your brain it is okay to stop, change, or rest. Please listen, it is OK to rest between heavy sets! You need to do this. BUT if that is all you ever do, if that is the only way you ever train, you will find yourself in a tough fight should things outside the weight room ever get rough!

Life happens outside of the weight room. It especially happens outside of the "health club." If we never teach ourselves how to sustain the ability to work, if we never teach ourselves how to maintain muscular effort for long periods of time, we are teaching ourselves how to quit or fail because life doesn't allow you to take a 5-minute rest break between heavy sets. Again, there is nothing wrong with traditional strength training. However, if you want to be strong enough to enjoy life and survive it, should you need to, then traditional strength training alone, will not help you. You need to do more.

Get this: if you lack the mental strength to "push" or fight when you need to the most, your body may lack the physical strength and ability to help you when you need it the most. The body will follow the mind. If your mind taps out in stressful situations, your body won't help you.

What about endurance athletes? Endurance athletes are no strangers to hard work. They also certainly know something or two about mental strength and fortitude. However, many endurance athletes fall short in their work capacity when it comes to manipulating more than their body from point (a) to point (b) because they neglect to incorporate strength training into their regimen. They sacrifice their absolute strength for their endurance. They develop the ability to run, bike, or swim for amazing distances, yet many of them are weak and incapable of staying on a task that requires any kind of full-body muscular exertion. They, too, are out of balance.

As the old saying goes, too much of anything can be a bad thing. What does it profit to be able to squat 800 pounds if you don't have the stamina to go for a 3-mile hike? Conversely, what does it profit to be able to run 26.2 miles in under 3 hours if you don't have the strength to carry a 50-pound suitcase across an airport without injuring your back?

We need a balance of strength. This balance of strength, this *"somewhere in the middle"* of the strength extremes, is really known as Work Capacity. Work capacity is the strength of an ox. It is having the ability to do "work", to stress the muscles through load, or resistance, and endure for a prolonged period of time. It is being able to relax and move under the stress of the task, the situation, or the event. Developing work capacity is how we learn to "make the hard things easy" and when we learn how to make the hard things easy, we get closer to becoming bulletproof.

Work Capacity

Today in the fitness world, "work capacity" is the new buzz word (yes, it is more than one word). Many people are touting it and "teaching" it, but I'm not sure they really get it. To make it even simpler than I explained above, work capacity is learning how to become comfortable with the uncomfortable. It's having the ability to perform work and endure for long periods of time. It is far greater than a physical attribute and it's also more than simple mental fortitude. It's also meditative; learning to have peace under fire, or stillness in distress, like the eye of a storm.

Before we dive into work capacity, I'd like to tell you about its father, John Brookfield. You may not know who he is, but you are probably familiar with his creation: The Battling Ropes System®. Many people don't know this, but Battling Ropes was first used inside the NFL and it grew from there. Now, the entire free world knows how to use a rope for exercise because of John Brookfield. He started the whole rope-exercise phenomenon. But that is just scratching John's surface. He is a modern-day Sampson, a man who knows no physical limit or mental constraint.

For example, when most people try to use ropes for training, they may be able to make steady waves at a wave-pace of 100 waves per minute for 30 seconds. With training, they may get up to a whole minute. Those that have trained under John eventually learn to perform the arduous task of making continuous waves for 20 whole minutes at a pace of 110 waves per minute. That is an amazing feat for any human. That is work capacity. But John can maintain 110 or more waves per minute for more than 2 continuous hours. Without stop. Recently, he told me that he was certain he could maintain that pace for 8 hours. He is right... Putting the Battling Ropes aside, John has also achieved multiple entries in the Guinness Book of World records for amazing feats, like dragging a 40,000-pound transfer trailer truck one mile in less than an hour; 50 minutes and 54 seconds to be exact...

As you can glean from this, John isn't human. Or he is superhuman, rather. He *is* work capacity, as strong as the ox, or stronger. He has learned to become very comfortable being very uncomfortable. Through doing this, he has learned to remove all limits from his mind and body. For John, one of the keys to doing this is training the body through training the mind. He sets his mind on a task and follows just one rule: Complete the task. He approaches this much like you would map a route with a smart phone by setting the coordinates and following the route, only you don't take potty breaks or lunch breaks. You simply drive until you get there.

John was and is a pivotal influence in my life. For whatever reason, he took me under his wing and taught me how to build a mind and body that will not stop. I'll be honest, in the beginning, I thought he was a crazy man. But now I know he is a brilliant genius who has learned that "all things are possible to him who believes."

Much of what I'm about to share with you are the lessons I've learned from John. You can become bulletproof by training to build tremendous work capacity: great absolute strength **and** great strength endurance. It all starts in your head. You just have to set your navigational system to get you where you want to go.

Calibrating Your GPS

Not so long ago, when the GPS (Global Positioning System) first came out, the way I traveled changed. I no longer needed a map. I could just plug in the address to where I wanted to go and my GPS would plan my route and tell me where and when to turn. It was great! When it worked...

Thank God for smart phones and map apps!

Anyway, sometimes my GPS would take me on routes that had dead ends, road blocks, heavy traffic, detours, pot holes, dirt roads, washed out roads, road construction, etc... In those days, my GPS did not care about what was going on along the route, it only cared to do its job: route me from where I was to where I wanted to go.

Like a route, life has obstacles along the way. There are bumps in the road, complete obstructions and seemingly dead ends. If we want to learn how to succeed and overcome in this life, we need to have the mindset of the GPS. We have to be single-minded in our focus so that we can get where we want to go.

We can learn how to develop this GPS mindset, this unrelenting resolve, through our physical training. We can do this by calibrating our GPS, our minds, and tell our body where we want it to go and how far we want it to go.

For example, imagine you wanted to spider-man crawl for half a mile without stopping. Half of a mile is a pretty good ways to spider-man crawl. Could you do it without taking a break, without letting your knees rest on the ground? Sure you can. Could you crawl a mile? Yes, you can. Can you imagine spider-man crawling a mile without stopping, without resting? You could do this if you set your mind on it. Ask me how I know...

If you think this is an insane task, and no one can do it, hopefully you will know how to do it before the end of this book. But know this: you can do it. In fact, you can pretty much do anything if you set your mind to it. Your parents were right when they told you that. The body and almost everything else follow the direction and lead of the mind.

I know this is silly but entertain me. What if you did learn how to do something crazy like crawl a mile nonstop? What if you developed the mental resolve and the physical fortitude to do something like that? What else might you be able to do? Anything. If you could do that, you would know that you could also do anything else you wanted to, you'd be strong enough to embrace all life's adventures.

Don't worry, you don't have to crawl a mile to be able to do anything. I'm only using it as an example. I do believe however that if you could spider-man crawl for 10 minutes nonstop you would still be able to do anything else you wanted to do. Just 10 minutes, but more about that later.

The point is, you can use your brain to make your body do what you want it to do. You just have to plug in the destination, be single minded, and stay the course.

Proverbs 23:7 says that "...As a man thinks in his heart, so is he." Simply put, your thoughts determine your outcome. If you think you can do something, you can do it. If you think you can't do something, you are also right.

You've probably heard the saying that "the body follows the head." It is true that physically where the head goes, the body will follow. That is the way we are physically "wired." But the same is also true for our minds: Where the mind goes, the body will follow. Your mind is your strongest muscle. If you exercise it, if you use it, you can make your body submit and follow where your mind will lead it.

The truth is your mind is already leading your body now. So what thoughts are you keeping?

Anyway, a key component to becoming strong and able is that you have to be an overcomer. You have to see yourself as being strong, you have to see yourself resilient and healthy. When you see a mountain, say, "I can climb that." When you see a rabbit, think, "I'll bet I could catch him if I tried." When you go to get out of bed in the morning, imagine how good your back is going to feel instead of how stiff or sore you think it will feel.

Being strong lives in your head. If you can believe you are going to be an overcomer, if you can believe you will have a resilient body full of grace, power and strength, then you will have it. Conversely, if you always see yourself sick, weak, injured and without hope, well, you will have that as well.

Don't forget this: The body goes where the head goes, both literally and metaphorically. Your thoughts and beliefs have as much to do with the state and health of your body as your actions do.

If you have a lot of negative junk in your head about your body, your abilities, or even your family genetics, get rid of it. Choose to believe something else. Choose to start thinking about how wonderfully made your body is. Choose to **know** that your body was meant to be strong, resilient and capable of doing anything. Choose to believe the truth: You are not weak. You are strong. You are not fragile. You are resilient. This is true. You might as well believe it.

This mental component of building strength is just as important as the physical component. When you decide that *you are going to be strong*, you will become strong. And that is good news. No matter what state you are in right now, you can become better. You can become stronger and more capable than you are. And it all starts in your head before you ever even engage in any physical activity.

Your beliefs about yourself are that powerful. So, make sure you're believing the right things. Calibrate your GPS properly and then go after your destination with determination and focus.

If you are still wondering why someone would want to train their mind to be like a GPS and their body to be as strong as an ox, it is because life is challenging. Life has change, twists and turns that will try to overcome you. Life has resistance. If you want to be "successful" or if you want your life to matter, you will meet resistance. Dead things have no problem floating down a stream, but life happens up stream. If you want to go up stream, you need to know how to swim against the current. Having the mental and physical strength to stand and endure against life's currents, or life's uncertainties, can be the difference between living or existing. Each of us was made to choose living so we all need to have the ability to endure stress, tension and fatigue. And we can endure; with enough strength for the day at hand, especially if we train to do so.

When you train, your body may tell your min "I'm tired. I need to stop." If you listen to your b probably stop or rest. However, if you ignore your body's p.. and keep your mind set on your predetermined plan of action, you can make your body follow. You will learn that being "tired" is just a feeling — your body still has energy and power to give. Remember, there is a hero inside of you; one that never dreams of defeat or quit, it only dreams of being able to save the day. That hero in you *is* you. These methods are simply a way to help you realize your potential.

Don't worry, this is a process. There is a progression to being able to do this. You should also know that I'm not talking about being reckless and ignoring your body or pushing yourself to the point of injury. I'm talking about training safely and intelligently while being able to override your body's attempts to rest and quit. The methods and movements in this book are suitable for anyone at any fitness level. They will also challenge anyone, at any fitness level.

Once you learn how to set your mind and you start to get a few small victories, you will understand how building mental strength can build physical strength. You will soon believe that there is nothing you cannot do. It all starts with a decision and one small step of action. Again, in case you missed it earlier, the smallest step of action you can make is simply keeping your tongue on the roof of your mouth. You can do that. Start there.

PREPARING TO FLY

"Before we get started, does anyone want to get out?"
— Steve Rogers, Captain America: Winter Soldier

Becoming bulletproof is a process of progressing simplicity. It is owning the fundamentals of movement and thought and then building upon them a little at a time. It is only guided by a few rules:

1) Start where you are.

2) Do what you can do.

3) Don't move into pain.

We all have a starting point. No matter how we move, no matter our physical limitations, no matter our beliefs, we all have a place we can start from. If we can breathe, we are good to go. With every day we are given, we have a brand-new starting point. Some days it may seem like we are much further than we were and other days it may seem as if we have fallen behind the line. It doesn't matter. Just start.

Having said that, we can all move and train within the boundaries of our thoughts and bodies. We may not be able to push past certain limits, but we can certainly work inside of them and up against them. We may not all have the endurance to crawl for five minutes, but we can all certainly endure until we cannot. We can all do *what we can*.

Yes, we do what we can, but we don't move into pain. This is of most importance! The notion of "no pain no gain" is one of the biggest training lies we must not believe. Training in pain and with pain will sabotage your efforts in becoming bulletproof. Pain changes everything. It changes how the body moves, it overrides normal neural sequences causing movement compensations. These compensations, if trained through, can undermine the foundation of the Three Pillars of Human Movement and this can lead to injury. Pain means stop. It doesn't mean keep going. Pain is also "real hurt." It is different than being uncomfortable. You can train through being uncomfortable, that is fine and that is what I'm going to ask you to do. But don't train through pain. Training through pain won't make you a superhero but it can keep you from becoming one. Got it?

If you set your mental GPS and you are determined to become bulletproof, these rules will get you there.

You should also know, along with these rules, I have two guiding principles that I believe will serve you well:

1) It feels good to feel good — Having a body that feels good, one that is strong as it needs to be and free to move where it wants, is priceless AND it feels amazing. But even better than that is having a body and a soul that feels good. When your mind and emotions are confident, content and at peace and you have a body capable of anything, it "feels" wonderful.

2) Make the hard things easy — If you learn how to make hard things easy, if your mind and body are strong,

everything in life becomes easier; from physical endeavors to work and life stress, they all just get easier to handle and nothing can weigh you down.

When I train, I try to stick to my two principles and allow them to guide me in the right direction. Does what I'm doing allow me to make hard things easier and will it allow me to feel good? Really what I'm asking is will this help me become bulletproof? If the answer is a resolute "yes" I continue on. If the answer is a "no" I can set it down. Make sense?

Ok, so how do we get started? The best place to begin is through owning the movements of your own body and then progressively challenging those movements through time and load. If John Brookfield taught me anything, it's that time and a challenging task is the greatest way to strengthen your mind and body. Let's address a challenging task first.

Perceived Effort

If you engage in the following training templates and routines, you're going to need a governor to know when the task is too easy and when the task is too hard. We want to become bulletproof by challenging ourselves, not crushing ourselves and not kidding ourselves.

To accomplish this, we are going to use an effort scale of 1 — 10, 1 being "It was so easy I did it sleeping," 10 being "it was so hard it almost killed me." Ideally, for our training we want to be in the 5-7 range. If while training your session was a three, that could mean you are not challenging yourself with adequate intensity, load or effort. If, however, you are rating your session as a 9, it may be that you need to lower your intensity, load or effort.

Along with this scale of perceived effort, I also want you to "use your tongue as a governor." What this means is if while training, you have to open your mouth and gasp for breath, use that as an indicator to take a quick rest so you can restore and recover your ability to breathe through your nose. Remember, your tongue is the rudder that guides the whole ship. If you ignore it as an indicator to rest, you will likely not be moving and training optimally. You *want* optimal strength and health. You do. Allow yourself the opportunity to achieve it and heed what your tongue is telling you. If it can't stay where it belongs and your mouth pops open for air, REST and RECOVER. Over time, as your cardiovascular system strengthens, you will have to rest less and less until you don't have to rest at all. When this happens, hard things become easy and you are unstoppable.

The Woes of Time

A set amount of time can be soul crushing when you are performing an uncomfortable task. Doing anything you don't enjoy makes time seem to last forever. Training when your mind is screaming for you to stop makes seconds seem like hours. I often joke to my clients that the style of training we do helps them understand dog years better. Only it's worse. Training like this really "messes" with your mind.

For example, if you were to use your mental GPS and set out to walk with a 50-pound bag, held in your arms like a load of fire wood, for 5 minutes before you could put it down, your mind may start to suffer because your arms may start to scream at you. You may try to look at your watch and discover you're only 30 seconds in. Things like that make your mind go nuts, until they don't…

John Brookfield is simply a master at things like this. He frequently uses various hour glasses to determine how long he will perform a task. He does this to strengthen his mind because an hour glass really only tells you two things: There is sand above, or all the sand is below. You really can't look at an hour glass dripping sand and know how much more time it will take for the sand to run out. This is a great way to torture the mind until you learn how to relax under the stress of what you are doing and let go of the time. This is how hard things eventually become easy.

But don't worry, that's what John does. You don't have to use an hour glass, unless you want to.

Mastering Movement

If you want to become bulletproof you must have the ability to move well. If you can't move well, you are likely to be more fragile than impervious because optimal movement is the key to moving with enduring strength. When we don't have the ability move well, the nervous system puts limitations on our bodies to keep us safe. Stiffness, tightness, reduced range of motion, weakness, slowness — they are all protective mechanisms placed on the body by the nervous system. When these protective mechanisms are in place AND we ignore them or try to override them, un-good things tend to happen.

The best way to learn to master the movements of your body is to have free, unrestricted access to moving your body. How do we get unrestricted access to moving our bodies? We deliberately and consistently move the way we were designed by engaging in the Three Pillars of Human movement. And, we do this with patience.

It took you three years of learning to move to build a very durable body as a child. It is okay if it takes you longer than four weeks to build one as an adult. But if you show up every day and move through the Three Pillars often, you will begin to remove any movement restrictions you might have. What you will begin to find is that your range of motion improves as does your ease and quality of motion. You may find that things that were once heavy just seem lighter. You may also discover that your ability to learn and control new movements just seems "to happen."

It gets really easy to learn how to control your body's movements and learn new movement skills when you don't have any movement restrictions or protective mechanisms in place. It is also emboldening when you start to learn that there is very little you cannot do. In other words, when the brakes come off your body, the brakes come off your life's potential. You begin to believe you are able and capable of handling whatever may come.

Mastering movement, which also means mastering strength, starts with establishing the Three Pillars of Human Movement. The pillars are your original strength, your movement foundation for all you are able to do. They are the keys to your health and resiliency. I highly encourage you to read *Pressing RESET* to fully understand how to establish your Original Strength, but until then here is a bare minimum Pressing RESET program to get you going.

Do This <u>Every</u> <u>SINGLE</u> <u>Day</u>...

1) Practice breathing deep into your belly with your tongue resting on the roof of your mouth for 5 minutes a day, 2 to 3 times per day. In the quest for Becoming Bulletproof, this is the best position to do this in:

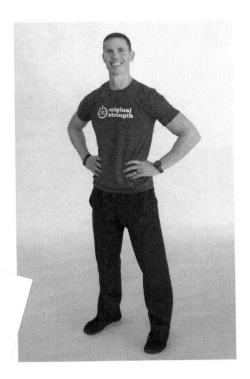

- Stand in this position.
- Place your tongue on the roof of your mouth and close your lips.
- Place your hands around your waist.
- Breathe in and out of your nose and pull air deep down into your belly.
    - Use your breath to try to spread and separate your fingers with your expanding belly and low back.
    - Try to feel your low back push your thumbs.

Don't make the mistake of dismissing how important proper breathing is. This is not just about getting air into your lungs. This is about building strength in your center. Your diaphragm is the chief stabilizing muscle in your inner core, it helps protect your spine. Reflexively stable spines are found in strong, well moving bodies. Also, do not dismiss this breathing position. It is powerful. Do it...

2) Practice head nods and head rotations for 2 minutes a day (1 minute for nods, 1 minute for rotations), 2 to 3 times per day. Use the same super position:

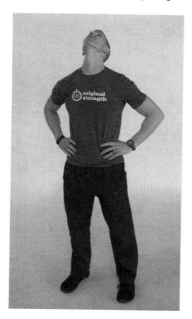

- Stand in this position.
- Place your tongue on the roof of your mouth and close your lips.
- Raise and lower your head as far as it will allow.
  - Lead the movement with your eyes.
  - When going into flexion, tuck your chin to your throat and flex the neck as far as it will go.
  - When moving into extension, hold the chin tuck until your head is level with the horizon.
- Do not hold your breath. Keep breathing through your nose.

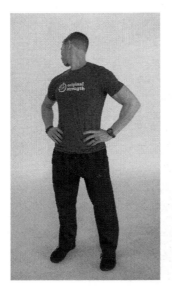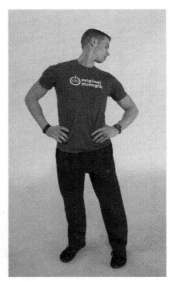

- Stand in this position.
- Place your tongue on the roof of your mouth and close your lips.
- Rotate your head left and right as if you are trying to look at your "back pockets."
- Lead the movement with your eyes.
- Do not drop your head. Look over your shoulders.
- Do not hold your breath. Keep breathing through your nose.

3) Practice rocking for 2 minutes, 2 to 3 times per day.

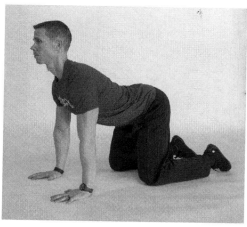

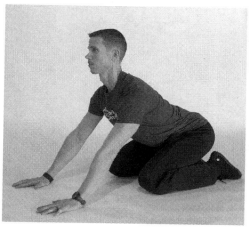

- Get on your hands and knees
- Keep your eyes and head up, level with the horizon.
- Keep your chest "proud" so that your back is "flat" like a silverback gorilla.
- Rock back and forth, rocking back as far as you can without losing your gorilla back.
- Explore feet plantar flexed (shoe laces down) and dorsiflexed (on the balls of your feet with the bottoms of your toes on the floor).

4) Cross-crawls for 1 minute, 2 to 3 times per day.

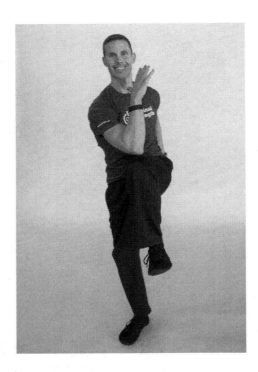

- Put your tongue on the roof of your mouth.
- Hold your head up and keep your eyes on the horizon.
- Keep a tall sternum. Be "proud" and hold a big chest.
- Touch your opposite limbs together.
- Can touch hand to thigh, elbow to knees, etc...

Do not dismiss this movement because of its simplicity! Cross-crawls can be quite miraculous. They are the easiest and most effective entry point that begins the restoration and strengthening of the nervous system. This movement can help rewire the brain, overcome learning disorders and set the body free to move and express itself.

This bare minimum RESET, these 10 minutes of movement two to three times per day, will help re-establish and solidify your Three Pillars of Human Movement. This can be done in the morning when you wake, before you engage in training, and even at night before you go to bed. If you perform this at night before bed, reverse the order. Start with cross-crawls, rocking, then head nods and rotations and finish with breathing.

Establishing your Original Strength by shoring up your Three Pillars is the beginning of becoming bulletproof and it is THE foundation for mastering and controlling the movements of your body.

#Strength10me

Ok, we know how to establish our foundation of strength and develop our mastery of movement. We know the three rules of becoming bulletproof and we know my guiding principles. We have a scale of perceived effort, we understand how to use the tongue to govern our rest breaks, and we know training under time has its woes. Great. But how do we set our GPS and lock in our desired coordinates and make our body submit to our mental intent?

We simply recall John Brookfield's one rule: Complete the task. For the training sessions in the Becoming Bulletproof Project the majority of our tasks will be performing movement for 10 minutes of time. There is nothing magic about staying on a task for ten minutes, but I have discovered for myself that if I can perform an uncomfortable task for 10 minutes, I can do it for 20, 30, or 40. It all feels the same after 10 minutes. I have tested this out, following John Brookfield's example, I have trained for 45 to 60 minutes while performing a task like spider-man crawling and I found 10 minutes to be the sweet spot. The level of uncomfortableness, or the level of "suck", remains much the same after 10 minutes. What this also conveys is that if you are "able" at 10 minutes, you are able at 20 minutes. To say this another way, if you are able to endure and withstand something unpleasant or even able to turn the unpleasant into your normal, then you are simply "able" — you can do anything. This may seem quite nebulous right now, but this will come to clarity for you once you begin this training.

You will discover your ability to endure and become. You will reach a knowing of "I have what it takes."

You might be thinking that doing anything for 10 minutes is beyond your ability, but do not worry. We are going to start where you are, and you are going to do what you can. Remember? In the beginning your task will be to complete ten minutes of **accumulated** movement. Using our perceived effort scale and your tongue as a governor, you are going to do what you can AND rest as you need to. As you become more capable and able, you'll find you have to rest less and less until you don't have to. You'll soon be able to complete ten minutes of **continuous** movement. Once you've done that, you'll be able to set your own GPS for 20, 40, 60 or more minutes of continuous movement, or whatever else you decide. Or, you'll be able to make the task more challenging by adding load, resistance or any other variable you want. The sky is the limit.

The other beautiful thing about training in 10-minute blocks is that it allows you to get done, or accomplish, what you can when you can. If your schedule demanded you break your training into 3 to 5 separate 10-minute sessions, you could absolutely do that AND still become bulletproof.

Strength, performance and ability are not about sets and reps. They are about showing up and putting in the time. Accumulating 10 minutes of work here and there adds up. Whether you complete 50 minutes of work at one time or you complete 50 minutes of work at 5 separate times in a day, 50 minutes of work done is 50 minutes of work done. That's a great day... Keep this in mind as you try to follow some of the training sessions below. You can make them fit into your day as you "see fit."

The Other Variables of Strength

Besides time, there are some other variables we can manipulate in order to challenge ourselves to get stronger. The first variable that comes to the minds of most is to use weight. Weight is great, but best when the body can easily and gracefully manage its own weight. Once bodyweight is mastered, adding more load to your frame is a sure way to build more strength, safely.

Another variable we can use to invite strength is resistance. Adding resistance to a movement is more than just adding a load, or weight. Adding resistance is purposefully hindering your ability to move or purposefully making your mind suffer.

One of my favorite non-time variables is distance. John Brookfield refers to it as distance covering. When using distance as a variable, your task is to cover a certain distance, depending on what you are doing and how you are doing it (all variables can play together if you are creative). For example, if you happen to find yourself at a soccer field with a 100-pound chain, you might set time aside and set your GPS on spider-man crawling while dragging the chain the length of the field 3 times. It takes how long it takes. You don't care. You just go, resting as needed, until you've covered the desired distance. Then you go home in victory. Job done. Covering distance is a great training variable.

The last variable I'll mention is speed. Adding speed, or reducing speed to a snail's pace, is another way to increase the challenge of whatever it is you are doing. Going fast takes energy and demands blood flow, while going painfully slow takes focus and demands control. Don't neglect the speed at which you move when you train; it matters. And don't use speed to cover up what you can't do well or to try to hurry through the task. If you don't own the movement you are performing, you need to do it super-slow until you do own it. Super-slow movement is another gateway to movement mastery, especially if the Three Pillars of Human Movement are being honored.

Whether you are using time, weight, resistance, speed, distance or a combination of all or any of them, remember the goal is to create a challenge for yourself on our effort scale somewhere between 5 to 7. I'm really okay with effort between 7 to 7.5 too, but that takes some fine tuning. For now, let's aim for 5 to 7!

Simple Movements

Aside from Pressing RESET and engaging in the Three Pillars of Human Movement, you really don't need a great deal of "movement know-how" when seeking to become bulletproof. It turns out that natural human movements like crawling, climbing and walking can go a very long way toward building an amazingly resilient body. In truth, all the body's natural movement patterns can be and should be used when seeking to build strength and health. The body was made to do these things:

- Push
- Pull
- Squat
- Hinge
- Roll
- Swing/Throw/Sling
- Get up and down from ground (a combination of all the movements listed above)
- Walk/Crawl/Climb/Carry/Jump

The programs to follow will use most, if not all of these movement patterns. If we engage often in the movements we are designed to make, we will be strong.

Having said that, the human body was ultimately designed to walk. Believe it or not, walking is the intended movement pattern designed to keep the nervous system healthy and it's the movement pattern designed to give strength to the body by keeping it tied together. We will do a great deal of loaded walking and carries throughout these programs. Loaded walking and carries should be a staple in your training. They are the "secret sauce" to building enduring strength. Done properly, they are very safe and yet they allow you to place awkward, unbalanced loads on the body. This is where strength is born. When the body learns how to reflexively manage off-centered, unbalanced, cumbersome loads on top of a foundation of Original Strength it becomes extremely strong and durable.

Simple Tools

The following tools are simply nice to have. They are not all necessary. Most of them are very affordable and most can be substituted for whatever you creatively come up with. Just because I list them doesn't mean you need them. These are simply the toys I like to have available.

- Backpack for loaded walking
  – Sandbags or weight of some type to load the bag with
- 50', 1.5" Battling Rope
- Large chain, or around 100 pounds of chain fashioned together (35', ½" chain works great)
- Two 5-gallon buckets
- Large rocks or kettlebells or dumbbells
- Sandbags or punching bags
- Indian Clubs — light 1 to 2 pound clubs, sticks, or hammers
- Sledge hammer or mace
  – Tire to accompany the hammer or mace
- Sled
  – Harness for dragging and pulling the sled
- Wheelbarrow
- Grass field — yes this is a nice-to-have tool/resource

Remember, these are "nice-to-haves." None of them are necessities, though I will be talking about them and using them in some of the following routines. If you have none of these, we just have to be more creative and that's great. Creativity ushers in discovery. If you've got a body, imagination and determination, we can move.

The Method

With all this talk about becoming bulletproof, building work capacity and getting comfortable with the uncomfortable, it might seem like we are setting ourselves up for some risky, if

ıgerous training. But that could not be further from the
. Safety, wisdom and simplicity are our main focus. All of
e qualities are inherently found in the natural movements
humans are designed to make but we will also be focusing on
low risk/high yield movements.

We are going to safely make ourselves uncomfortable to
reveal our strength. Anything that requires a great deal of
technical skill, anything that places undo stress on the body,
anything that is "risky" or has a large risk-to-reward ratio, we
aren't doing that!

In other words, we aren't participating in "exercise." Exercise
is a manmade solution to a manmade problem: not moving.
But exercise is the wrong solution. Moving by and through our
design is the right solution, especially if we want to become
bulletproof and truly discover our superpowers.

Ok, are you ready to move?

THE BECOMING BULLETPROOF TEMPLATE

"He's not a human. He's like a piece of iron."
— Ivan Drago, *Rocky IV*

Here is where we put it all together. We establish our Original Strength, we set our GPS, and we build our work capacity through our effort, natural human movements, and accumulated time. This is where we learn to get comfortable being uncomfortable and we begin to take flight.

As I mentioned above, I find doing tasks in 10-minute blocks to be extremely effective in developing enduring strength and physical resiliency. A Becoming Bulletproof routine is a routine where I string together three to six 10-minute tasks, depending on the individual's goals, time and abilities. In order to do this, there are certain tasks that need to be built up. In other words, you have to develop a certain level of work capacity to even be able to do these routines. This is simple to do, it just takes time and determination.

In the beginning, developing the capacity to perform these tasks can, in itself, be the training routine of the day. And that's ok. We've got a journey to embark on and embrace. We are not using teleportation or snapping our fingers to make this happen and we aren't trying to "hack" our body. We are trying to build our bodies the right way, on a solid foundation that can support everything we ever want to be able to do. Short cuts tend to undermine the foundation. That's not the way...

Below, I am going to list foundational tasks and abilities I think you need to have in your toolbelt. These abilities lend themselves well to creating fantastic movement sessions.

The Tasks at Hand

Be Able to Press RESET x 10 minutes

Why?

This establishes and ensures your Three Pillars of Human Movement are firmly in place. What this means is that your nervous system is healthy because you will be feeding it with optimal sensory input teaching your body how to stabilize, mobilize and express itself efficiently through all situations. In other words, it removes the limits from your body and reduces your chance of injury while also increasing your ability to build strength. This alone, if you did nothing else in this book, could eventually make you bulletproof. But it's too easy, so most wouldn't dare take me up on that... But you will do this as part of the Becoming Bulletproof Template. From here forward, there is one non-negotiable requirement. Deal?

How?

Press RESET every day for 10 minutes. If you are going to train, do it before you train. If you are not training on a particular day, still Press RESET. Do this every single day. You can use the routine outlined above or you can create your own from reading the *Pressing RESET* book or even stringing together the "movement snax" from the Original Strength YouTube[3] page. This is your first 10-minute task!

What tools do you need?

- Your body
- Floor space
- A stopwatch

Be Able to Perform Battling Ropes Waves (Velocity Training) x 10 minutes without stop

Why?

?? If you have the will to work up to and master 10 minutes of continuous waves you will learn how to relax under stress; how to push through extreme levels of discomfort and even moments of fear. This is because velocity training (wave training) with ropes demands much from the mind and the lungs. It creates a special stress that makes both the brain and body plead to stop. The body is never in danger, but the physical demand placed on the body is ferocious. The intensity of velocity training places a huge demand on the mind, pushing it to a "panic-like" state. If the mind learns to relax through this, the body's endurance limits are removed.

Remember, the body follows the head (the mind). That is the way we are designed. If you want to push your body beyond limits and become bulletproof, you need to lead the way with your mind. Velocity training, especially when combined with managing and maintaining **nasal, diaphragmatic** breathing is the essence of being bulletproof. It is a demonstration of superior strength, power, endurance and mental tenacity. That's right. Your goal, if you choose to tackle this task, is to accomplish this with your mouth closed, keeping your tongue on the roof of your mouth and breathing deep into your lungs through your nose. You can do this. Even if it seems impossible. When you do accomplish this, you will believe that you can do anything. That's a valuable belief...

What tools do you need?

- 50', 1.5" rope
- Metronome
- Stopwatch
- Anchor point to attach rope to
- Place to stand

How?

Velocity training is best approached one wave at a time. In keeping with the rules laid out earlier, we are going to start where we are and do what we can. If you need to stop, you stop. If your mouth pops open to breathe, you stop. When you recover, you continue on. It's pretty simple. But here is an outline for you:

1) Set your rope up by attaching it to an anchor point.

2) Set the metronome to 80 bpm for 2-handed waves (parallel waves) or 160 bpm for alternating waves.

3) Get your stopwatch ready so you can time how long you can maintain this pace.

4) Grasp both ends of the rope with an underhanded grip.

5) Stand so that the rope is not taunt (tight).

   - When you grasp both ends of the rope walk the rope back so that it is tight.
   - Once the rope is stretched completely out and its tight, take a step forward allowing the rope to sag towards the floor.
   - You want slack in the rope to run the waves through it...

6) With your lips shut, so that you are only breathing through your nose, match the metronome with your waves.

   - The waves should travel all the way to the anchor point.

7) Start the watch when you start your waves ON pace.

8) IF your mouth pops open to breathe, stop your waves and the stopwatch. Note the time.

9) IF you lose pace with the metronome, stop your waves and the stopwatch. Note the time.

10) IF your waves no longer reach the anchor point, stop your waves and the stopwatch. Note the time.

11) IF you simply stop from burnout, stop the watch and note the time.

12) Use a 1:1 work to rest ratio if you can make waves for up to two minutes.

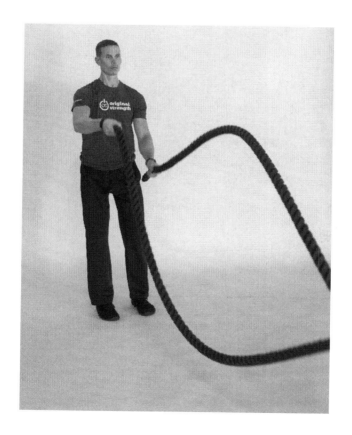

13) Accumulate 10 minutes of work (waves). This may take 30 minutes. That's great!

- For example, 30 seconds of waves/30 seconds of rest x 20 rounds = 10 minutes of work done in 20 minutes.

14) Once you can maintain waves for more than two minutes, use a 1-minute recovery time between rounds.

This is a crude way to go about this, but if you follow the rules and set your GPS, you can "easily" accomplish this task. If you need a more structured program for this feat, I have a very specific 10-minutes of Velocity training program available online. You can find that here:

OSi-Online.com

If you follow the outline above two to three times per week, you will accomplish your 10 minutes of continuous waves in a few weeks. You'll discover new progress every time you engage in this task; as you become more capable from day to day, your waves will last longer, and you'll recover faster, having to rest less and less until you don't have to rest at all. It's a pretty awesome accomplishment.

Be Able to Leopard Crawl x 10 minutes without stop

[Why?]*!
Crawling strengthens everything about you; your mind, your nervous system, your sensory systems, your ENTIRE body. Crawling for long periods of time really works on the mind because it becomes very uncomfortable. Time seems to stand still while the muscles start to ache as the heart rate and breathing rate rapidly increase as if you're running wind sprints. It's an all out assault on the body. What seems so childish and simple ends up being so, well, hard. It's hard and it just sucks. Until it doesn't.

The great thing about crawling is that even though it seems like torture, it actually continues to nourish the nervous system and every step you take increases reflexive strength and stability — every step increases and builds your Original Strength and makes you more bulletproof. If you pass on the 10 minutes of Battling Ropes (and you shouldn't), DO NOT PASS on this.

As brutal as crawling for time is, eventually as the mind and body get stronger, crawling just gets easier and easier. Ten minutes of crawling eventually feels like 1 minute and 30 minutes of crawling feels just like 10 minutes. And just in case you are wondering, a person that can leopard crawl for 10 minutes can just about do ANYTHING they want to do. That alone removes most all limits. The only thing better than leopard crawling for 10 minutes is backwards leopard crawling for 10 minutes!

What tools do you need?

- Stopwatch
- Possibly knee pads
- Space to move

How?

Ok, it may be best to tackle this task in stages:

Stage1: Crawling on the Hands and Knees for 10 minutes

1) Get on your hands and knees (wear knee pads if needed) and crawl forward.

2) Start your watch when you begin crawling. Stop your watch when/if you need to rest.

3) Keep your head held up and your eyes on the horizon.

4) Make sure your opposite limbs are moving together. Example: Right arm moves with left leg...

5) Keep your lips shut and maintain diaphragmatic breathing.

6) Accumulate 10 minutes of crawling.

- If your mouth pops open to breathe, rest and stop the clock.
- Resume the clock once you can continue crawling with your lips shut.

7) Once you can accomplish 10 uninterrupted minutes of crawling, continue to Stage 2.

Stage 2: Leopard Crawling for 10 minutes
1) Get on your hands and feet and leopard crawl forward.

- In leopard crawling, the knees track under the torso, inside of the elbows.

2) Start your watch when you begin crawling. Stop your watch when/if you need to rest.

3) Keep your head held up and your eyes on the horizon.

4) Keep your chest "tall" and your butt held down, below your head.

5) Make sure your opposite limbs are moving together. Example: Right arm moves with left leg…

6) Keep your lips shut and maintain diaphragmatic breathing.

7) Accumulate 10 minutes of leopard crawling.

- If your mouth pops open to breathe, rest and stop the clock.
- If your head drops and your butt pops up above your head, rest and stop the clock.
- Resume the clock once you can continue crawling with your lips shut and keep your butt down.

8) Once you can accomplish 10 uninterrupted minutes of leopard crawling, continue to Stage 3.

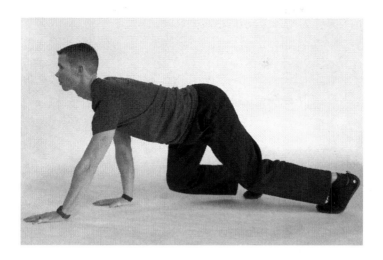

Stage 3: You can do whatever you want to do — you're strong enough. But, try this backwards!

Be able to "Climb a Mountain" of Squats and Pushups in under 20 minutes

There are always exceptions to the rules. Not everything has to be in 10-minute blocks. There are some tasks that lend themselves well to becoming bulletproof due to their difficulty. Whenever I combine movements like squats and pushups, I like to open up the time frame and accomplish a non-time limiting task. When climbing a mountain, the task is to complete climbing up from 1 to 10 reps of each movement and then climb back down from 10 to 1 of each movement. This gives 100 reps of each movement. That's a fairly good task to complete in 20 minutes or less; especially if you can climb up and down the entire mountain while maintaining nasal breathing!

Why?

This builds a tremendous base of strength and mental tenacity. It is also easily measurable and it reveals progress being achieved. The stronger you become, the higher you can climb or the faster you can complete your mountain.

What tools do you need?
- Stopwatch
- Potentially a weight of some type (dumbbell, kettlebell, sandbag, rock, llama, etc)
- Potentially a weight vest

How?

1) Pick two movements. Here, we are choosing squats and pushups.

   - Squats can be bodyweight, or you can hold a weight in front of your chest (dumbbell, kettlebell, sandbag, rock, small child, etc.)
   - Pushups can be bodyweight, or you can make them harder by elevating feet or wearing a weight vest.

2) Perform 1 squat, then 1 pushup. Then perform 2 squats, then 2 pushups. 3&3, 4&4..., 9&9, 10&10, 9&9, 8&8, 7&7...1&1.

   - You add one repetition every time you come back to the first movement until you reach 10 of each. Then you subtract one repetition every time you come back to the first movement until you reach 1 of each.
   - You will only perform 10 reps of each ONCE.

3) Start your stopwatch once you begin climbing the mountain.

   - You are going to let the clock run. Do not stop the clock if you stop to rest, though rest as you need to.

4) Record the entire time it takes you to climb your mountain.

5) The goal is to get 100 reps of each movement in 20 minutes or less.

   - Once accomplished, this is easy to progress by holding weight or increasing weight.

- This can also be done with whichever movements you want to pair like, burpees and pull-ups, pushups and deadbugs, "light" deadlifts and presses, etc.

Be able to perform the Weight of Water x 10 minutes without stop

The Weight of Water is perhaps the most brilliant training task John Brookfield has ever dreamed up. I believe it's even more ingenious than battling ropes. On its simplest execution, you position yourself in a plank on your hands in between two buckets, one full of water and one empty. You take a small cup and attempt to empty the one bucket and fill the other bucket WHILE you hold yourself up in that plank. Oh, and you are not allowed to spill the water. You have to focus. Yeah...

Why?

This drill is priceless when it comes to learning about yourself, your will, and your faith. Faith? Yes, this drill is brutal, and it will test you. You may find you've been transferring water for 8 minutes with no discernible change in the water level of your bucket. This can be soul crushing, especially if your intention is to finish emptying the entire bucket. I'm only asking you for 10 minutes here but emptying a bucket and filling the other could easily take 30 minutes or more depending on the size of your transfer cup. Having said that, emptying a bucket will teach you that you can indeed do anything. If you can maintain a plank for that long, never putting a knee down, your mind, your will, and your body will not break. You're unstoppable and you know it.

What tools do you need?

- Two 5-gallon buckets
- Water
- A small cup (1 oz to 6 oz)

How?

1) Fill one 5-gallon bucket with water and keep one empty.

2) Place the buckets 2 — 3 feet apart.

3) With your small cup, position yourself between the buckets and assume a pushup / plank position on your hands.

4) Start your stopwatch once you position yourself between the buckets.

5) Take the small cup and fill it by dipping it into the bucket with water.

6) Place the small cup full of water on the floor underneath you.

7) Grab the cup with your other hand and empty its contents into the empty bucket.

8) Place the empty cup on the floor underneath you and repeat this process.

   • The cup always returns to the floor after it is filled or emptied.

9) DO NOT SPILL THE WATER. Concentrate.

10) Keep your lips shut and breathe through your nose.

11) Accumulate 10 minutes of water transfer without coming down from the plank position.

   • If you rest, stop the clock.
   • If your mouth pops open to breathe, rest.
   • If your butt pops way up in the air and your plank looks like an triangle, rest.
   • When you can resume, start the clock back.

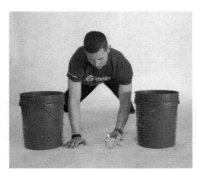 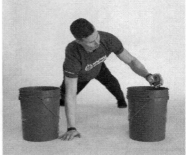

Be able to jump rope x 10 minutes without stop

Why?

This is just a great, simple task to be able to perform. It lends itself well to building mental and physical stamina especially when performed through nasal breathing and it teaches coordination and timing.

What tools do I need?

- A "fast" jump rope. The rope needs to be able to spin at high rpms.
- An open-faced clock with a minute hand.
  – Or a stopwatch

How?

1) If using the clock, start jumping when the minute hand is on 12.

2) Try to achieve a pace between 130 to 150 jumps per minute.

   - You'll have to count that, and you'll have to be able to count fast.

3) Keep your lips shut and breathe through your nose.

4) Accumulate 10 total minutes of jumping rope.

   - If your mouth pops open to breathe, rest and stop the clock.
   - Resume when you can manage your breath and start the clock.

5) If you trip over the rope, as expediently as you can, continue jumping and don't sweat it.

6) Work your way to 10 straight minutes.

Again, being able to perform this collection of tasks is a great way to build a foundation that allows you to create some unique and uncomfortable training sessions that will build a mind of iron and body of steel. You don't have to accomplish them all, but you can. The journey to accomplishing any of these tasks can make you bulletproof on their own. But as you accomplish each one, you'll continue to "harden" yourself and elevate your confidence in your ability. You just know *that you know* you can do anything, and you have no limits. In other words, the superhero inside you knows you are.

Other Non-Time Limited Honorable Tasks

The following tasks are also formidable and rewarding. In truth, they are actually training sessions in and of themselves. They too will put you well on your way to becoming bulletproof. I list them here because they can require a great deal of planning, and they may require that you have access to a track or a field. However, if you are determined, you can do most of these in your neighborhood or through your neighbors' yards. With all of these tasks, work to maintain nasal breathing and steady movement.

- Leopard Crawl a quarter of a mile around a track.
  – Rest as you need to but try not to need to.

- Backwards Leopard Crawl a quarter of a mile around a track.
  – Rest as you need to. One day you won't need to.

- Crawl the length of a football field forward and then backward for two round trips.
  – Rest as you need to.

- Crawl while dragging 100 pounds of weight (chains, sled, sandbags, etc.) the length of a football field forward then backward. Then go home.
  Depending on how you drag the weight, attached to your body or by using your hands, this can be quite humbling and empowering.

– The ways to drag a load while crawling across a field are quite numerous. If you have an imagination, you'll have more than enough to explore for years.

- Push a weighted sled, the length of a football field for 2 to 3 round trips or for time.

- Drag a weighted sled, the length of a football field for 2 to 3 round trips.

- Carry a very heavy sandbag in your arms like a load of fire wood the length of a football field for a certain number of trips or for time.
  – Put the bag down on the ends of the field and shake it out. Resume when able.

- Lunge or "long stride" the length of a football field for a certain number of trips.
  – This can be done as a bodyweight movement or you can attach or hold a load of some type.

- Leopard Crawl while pushing a heavy slam ball, rock, or sled across the length of a football field then pull it with you as you leopard crawl back backward. Then go home.

- Walk through your neighborhood with a wheelbarrow full of anything you can put in it.
  – Make your wheelbarrow heavy and walk for time (30 minutes is good).
  – Rest as you need to.
  – Find some good hills.

The Bulletproof Sessions

The following sessions are how I train myself and my clients. Remember, in order to embrace this method, you'll need to let go of your thoughts on exercise. We aren't exercising here, we are moving in and through our design. Some of these sessions may seem impossible, but I guarantee you that one day they will become easy and ordinary to you. Through this experience you will know how the hard things become easy.

These sessions are also just **ideas** and examples. You may have to take them and fit them into your schedule and your needs and goals. You may even have to be creative about how you fit them into your day. The beautiful thing about training in 10-minute blocks is that it all adds up. You can train in small 10-minute sessions throughout your day — if you need to.

Having said all of that, I'll try to provide some "loose" structure and direction as we go...

Beginner Sessions

Tackle and master the Tasks above. And, be patient and enjoy the process.

Here are some examples of what this may look like as you progress:

Example 1

Mondays and Thursdays

- Press RESET x 10 minutes.

- Climb a Mountain with Squats and Pushups — complete the task and record how long it takes you. If you have to break up your pushups, or do them on your knees, do it. If you have to take 100 rest breaks, do it. Do what you can. Rest as you need to. Conquer your mountain.
  - IF this takes you longer than 20 minutes, you are done for the day.

- IF you can complete this mountain in 20 minutes or less, perform **Chest Carries** x 10 minutes — You'll need a weight of some type (kettlebell, dumbbell, sandbag, etc)
  - men: 30 to 50 pounds, women: 20 to 40 pounds
  - Keeping a tall chest, squat or hinge down to pick up the weight, stand and hold it in front of your chest.

- Walk 10 yards with the weight then put it down.
- Turn around, pick the weight back up and then walk back.
- Repeat this over and over for 10 minutes.
- Rest as you need to.
- Keep your tongue on the roof of your mouth and breathe through your nose.
- Note: it is possible to pick up the weight more than 40 times (that would be moving 2000 pounds if you used a 50-pound weight) and travel more than 4 football fields during these 10 minutes. That's good work…

Tuesdays and Fridays

- Press RESET x 10 minutes

- Battling Ropes for 10 minutes of accumulated work done.
  - If this takes you longer than 20 minutes, you are done for the day.

- If you accomplish this in 10 to 20 minutes, go for a **Ruck Walk** x 20 minutes.
  - Get your backpack and fill it with "soft" weight. Bags of sand work great here.
  - The pack need not weigh more than 25 pounds.
  - Cinch the shoulder straps close together to pull them out of the crease in your shoulders.
  - Walk with purpose, as if you are in a hurry, by swinging your arms FROM YOUR SHOULDERS.
    - Your shoulder swing should match your hip swing.
  - Keep your lips shut and breathe through your nose.
  - If your mouth pops open to breathe, stop and rest.
    - Resume when you can return to nasal breathing.
  - Accumulate 20 minutes of walking.

Wednesdays and Saturdays

- Press RESET x 10 minutes

- Leopard Crawl x 10 minutes
  - If this takes around 20 minutes to complete, good job, you're done for the day.

- If you complete this in 10 minutes, good job, perform **Suitcase Carries** x 10 minutes.
  - Men: grab a weight between 40 to 70 pounds, women: grab a weight between 30 to 50 pounds.
    - Ideally you want the weight to be heavy enough to accrue yourself a fine if you were trying to take it on an airplane.
  - Grab the weight in your right hand, hold it by your side and walk for 15 yards, turn around and come back.
  - Set the weight down, pick it up in your left hand, hold it by your side and walk for 15 yards, turn around and come back.
  - Repeat this over and over until 10 minutes expires on the clock.
  - Keep your mouth closed and keep your tongue on the roof of your mouth.

Sundays = REST

Example 2

Mondays

- Press RESET x 10 minutes

- Climb a Mountain of squats and pull-ups x 10 minutes
  - Climb as high as you can, don't stop at 10 if you get that far.
  - Record how high you get at 10 minutes

- Weight of Water x 10 minutes

Tuesdays

- Press RESET x 10 minutes
- Suitcase Carry x 10 minutes (as outlined above)
- Backward Leopard Crawl x 10 minutes

Wednesdays

- Press RESET x 10 minutes
- Ruck Walk with weighted backpack x 30 minutes (as outlined above)

Thursdays

- Press RESET x 10 minutes

- Weight of Water
  - Use a 6 oz cup.
  - Empty the entire bucket and fill the other.
  - It takes how long it takes, and GREAT JOB!

Fridays

- Press RESET x 10 minutes
- Chest Carry x 10 minutes (as outlined above)
- Forward Leopard Crawl x 10 minutes

Saturdays

- Press RESET x 10 minutes
- Ruck Walk with weighted backpack x 30 minutes (as outlined above)

Sundays = Fun days!

- Enjoy yourself and your family!

These aren't rigid sessions, they are examples of what a beginning bulletproof session may look like. You can follow these exactly or you can "get the idea" and create your own. Either way, if you put in the work, you'll get stronger, start to

ɹetter, and you'll begin learning how hard things become
y. Then, you'll be ready for more advanced training sessions.

Intermediate to Advanced Becoming Bulletproof Sessions

When you can routinely tackle and complete any of the tasks
mentioned above with ease, you are ready for more advanced
training sessions. This is where you develop work capacity,
mental tenacity, and physical resiliency with no real limits.
All the brakes come off here; you're inner hero is revealed and
you are prepared and able to withstand life's events. I know
it sounds crazy, but if you get to this point, you'll absolutely
know what I am talking about. Here are some examples of
what these more advanced sessions may look like:

Example 1:

Mondays and Thursdays

- Press RESET x 10 minutes

- Climb a Mountain of Goblet Squats and Pushups —
  Use a weight to hold in front of your chest. Climb all the
  way up to 10 of each and then back down to 1 of each.
  Complete the mountain.
  – Ideally you can complete this in 15 to 18 minutes though
    it doesn't matter if it takes longer. Just keep moving.

- Leopard Crawl nonstop x 10 minutes

- Chest Carries x 10 minutes — see above in beginner's
  example

- March and Cross-Crawl Walk x 10 minutes
  – March 20 yards
      – Spread your fingers wide and swing your arms
        from your shoulders
      – Land on the balls of your feet. Do not land on
        your heals.

- After you march 20 yards, turn around and walk back while performing Cross-Crawls
  - Walk back touching opposite arm to leg as you walk back.
  - Touch where you can; elbow to knee, forearm to thigh, hand to leg...

Tuesdays and Fridays

- Press RESET x 10 minutes

- Sled Work x 10 minutes (you'll need a sled you can push)
  - Attach a battling rope to a sled with 200 pounds on it
    - Weight doesn't matter as much as friction. You want enough friction to make this a challenge of 5 to 7 on our effort scale.
  - Straighten the rope all the way out.
  - Pull the sled to you, keeping your chest up.
  - When the sled has reached you, run it back to where you pulled it from.
  - THEN Backward Leopard Crawl to the far end of the rope.
  - Repeat this over and over for 10 minutes.

- Sledge Hammer / Mace Work x 10 minutes (you'll need a hammer or mace and a tire -it's worth it)
  - Square up on a tire, swing your mace (10 — 15 pounds is great) from side to side striking the tire.
  - You are alternating sides with each swing working the "X" (your body is the X).
  - After 20 hits, get to your hands and feet and perform 20 elevated Cross-Crawl touches.
  - It's like you are in the Leopard Crawl Position and you are performing cross-crawls....
  - After your 20 touches, return to hitting the tire.
  - Work this back and forth for 10 minutes.
  - Rest as you need to and have fun.

- Ruck Walk x 20 minutes
  - Remember to walk with purpose, as if you are in a hurry.
  - Swing those shoulders…

Wednesdays and Saturdays

- Press RESET x 10 minutes
- Jump rope x 10 minutes nonstop
- Battling ropes x 10 minutes nonstop
- Backward Leopard Crawl in slow motion x 10 minutes nonstop
  - Crawl slow enough to makes sloths jealous.

Sundays — find an adventure

Example 2:

Mondays and Thursdays (you'll need a sandbag)

- Press RESET x 10 minutes

- Backward Leopard Crawl while dragging a "heavy" sandbag x 10 minutes
  - Backward Leopard Crawl x 20 yards while pulling your sandbag with you along the way.
    - Get on your hands and feet behind your sandbag.
    - Reach forward, grab your bag, pull it toward you, then crawl backward a few steps.
    - Reach forward with your other hand, grab your bag, pull it toward you, then crawl backward a few steps.
    - Alternate hands with every pull.
  - Keep your butt down.
  - When you have traveled 20 yards, standup, shoulder the bag and walk back to where you started.
  - Then repeat the process.
  - When you walk back with the bag again, shoulder it on the other shoulder…
  - Try to move the entire 10 minutes without rest

- Sandbag getups x 10 minutes
    - Grab a "heavy" sandbag and place it on your shoulder
        - Imagine the sandbag is a big, heavy child that you do not want to drop.
    - Lie down with your sandbag on your shoulder.
        - Don't drop your baby.
        - You can lie down how you want.
    - Get up with it.
    - Try for 3 reps each side before switching sides.
    - Repeat this for 10 minutes.
    - Strive for constant movement but rest as you need to.

- Suitcase Carries x 10 minutes — see outline above
    - Make it a "heavy" suitcase

- Brisk Walk with Indian Clubs x 10 minutes
    - Grab a pair of Indian Clubs or two small hammers.
    - Walk with purpose, as if you are late for a hot date.
    - Swing your shoulders to match your hips.
    - Keep your eyes on the horizon.
    - Keep your lips shut and breathe through your nose.

Tuesdays and Fridays

- Press RESET x 10 minutes

- Sled Work x 10 minutes
    - Make the sled "heavy."
        - Again, it's more about friction. We want an effort level around a 7 on our scale of 1 to 10.
    - Get a TRX strap or a harness and hook to one end of sled.
    - Drag the sled backward 20 yards as if dragging a deer out of the woods or a tarp of leaves out to the road for pick up.
    - Then push the sled back to where you started.
    - Repeat this back and forth for 10 minutes.
    - Try for constant movement with nasal breathing.

- Shoulder Carries x 10 minutes
  - Grab a heavy bag and place it on your right shoulder.
  - Walk for 15 yards and put it down.
  - Pick it up and place it on your left shoulder
  - Walk back to where you started.
  - Repeat this until 10 minutes has expired

- Ruck Walk x 20 minutes
  - Use between 25 to 35 pounds in your pack.
  - Walk like you mean it.

Wednesdays and Saturdays — at the field, with a chain

- Forward Leopard Crawl while dragging a chain
  - Go to a football or soccer field
  - Drag a 100-pound chain, or sled, or sandbag as you Leopard Crawl the length of the field.
  - Put on a harness and attach it to whatever you are dragging.
  - Leopard Crawl the length of the field.
  - Rest.
  - Leopard Crawl back to where you started.
  - Go home.

Sundays — reminisce about crawling at the field

<u>Example 3</u>

Mondays

- Press RESET x 10 minutes

- Lateral Leopard Crawl on your hands and feet x 20 minutes
  - Crawl sideways to your right for 20 yards
  - Crawl sideways to your left for 20 yards
  - Repeat over and over for 20 minutes
  - Try not to put a knee down and keep moving.
  - Breathe through your nose.

Tuesdays

- Press RESET x 10 minutes

- Sled work x 30 minutes
  - You'll need a rope, a sled, a weight (I'm using a 24K kettlebell in this example)
  - Attach a battling rope to a sled with 200 pounds on it
    - Remember, weight doesn't matter as much as friction. You want enough friction to make this a challenge of 5 to 7 on our effort scale.
  - Straighten the rope all the way out.
  - Place the weight (my 24K kettlebell) near / beside the end of the rope.
  - With the kettlebell, perform 10 goblet squats (squat 10 times while holding the bell in front of your chest)
  - Put the bell down and pick up the end of the rope.
  - Make 20 waves with the rope.
    - The waves should travel the entire distance to the sled — 50 ft.
  - Pull the sled to you, keeping your chest up.
  - When the sled has reached you, run it back to its starting point.
  - THEN backward Leopard Crawl back to the end of the rope.
  - Repeat this sequence over and over for 30 minutes: 10 squats, 20 waves, pull the sled, push the sled, crawl backward…
  - Strive for 30 minutes of constant movement.
  - You can do it.

Wednesdays — Heavy Carry Day

- Press RESET x 10 minutes
- Chest Carries x 10 minutes
- Shoulder Carries x 10 minutes
- Suitcase Carries x 10 minutes
- Overhead Carries x 10 minutes

- Carry what you like: a bar, a plate, a sandbag, a slosh pipe, a kettlebell, a dumbbell, a dog, etc…
  - If carrying a dumbbell or kettlebell, carry only ONE for unilateral carries.
  - If carrying a slosh pipe or dog, focus at all times.
- Let's use a 45 pound plate…
- Grab the plate like a steering wheel and press it overhead.
- Walk for 20 yards.
- Lower the plate and wisely place it on the floor.
- Turn around and pick the plate back up and press it overhead.
- Walk back to your starting point.
- Repeat this over and over for 10 minutes.

Thursdays

- Press RESET x 10 minutes
- John Brookfield's Infinity Crawl x 20 minutes
  - Get two 5-gallon buckets or foam rollers and place them 3 feet apart.
  - Get on your hands and feet and Backward Leopard Crawl around the buckets
    - Serpentine your body around the buckets, tracing infinity symbols around the buckets.
  - Keep your head up and look over your shoulders to find the buckets. Don't look for them by dropping your head.
  - Keep your butt down below your head.
  - Keep your lips shut and breathe through your nose.
  - You're welcome.

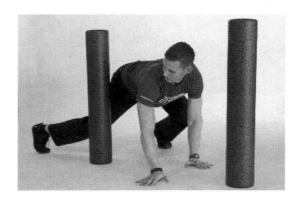

Fridays

- Press RESET x 10 minutes

- Sled work x 30 minutes
  - You'll need a rope, a sled, harness or TRX type equipment
  - Attach a battling rope to a sled with 200 pounds on it
    - Remember, weight doesn't matter as much as friction. You want enough friction to make this a challenge of 5 to 7 on our effort scale.
    - Attach the harness or TRX to the other end of the sled.
  - Straighten the rope all the way out.
  - Perform 10 pushups.
  - Stand up and pick up the end of the rope.
  - Make 10 waves with your right hand and then 10 waves with your left hand.
    - The waves should travel the entire distance to the sled — 50 ft.
  - Pull the sled to you, keeping your chest up.
  - When the sled has reached you, grab the harness or TRX and drag the sled back to where you started.
  - THEN March back to the end of the rope.
    - March as if the ground is hot; fast feet.
    - Spread your fingers and swing your shoulders.
  - Repeat this sequence over and over for 30 minutes: 10 pushups, 10 waves right, 10 waves left, pull the sled, drag the sled, march...
  - Strive for 30 minutes of constant movement.
  - You can do it.

Saturdays — Conditioning Fun

- Press RESET x 10 minutes

- Jump rope x 10 minutes

- Battling Ropes x 10 minutes

- Hit the tire with your mace or sledge hammer x 10 minutes
  – Strive for 10 minutes of constant hits (around 300 hits at a good pace)
- Leopard Crawl and skip x 10 minutes
  – Leopard Crawl 20 yards
  – Skip back to where you started
  – Repeat for 10 minutes...

Again, these Bulletproof Sessions are EXAMPLES of what this type of training may look like. This is how I have trained and how I have learned. The above examples may work great for you, but you may also need to determine what works best for you given your resources and your current goals.

This type of training fit my schedule and my needs. I simply wanted to be Superman, so I laid down conventional means — things I had always done for years — and found a different way. Or truly, it found me. Either way, I did let go of some old notions and old methods in order to fully embrace this type of training. You may have to do this as well, if you haven't.

Springs and Slings

The tasks and training sessions above are almost perfect for making yourself bulletproof. Almost. There is one small area we could address or add to make the becoming bulletproof journey more perfect. We need to address the springs and slings.

We are also made to bounce and leap. We have springs that help us hop and we have slings that propel us from one place to the other. It may help to think as your springs being your legs and as your slings being your torso. In order to become bulletproof and remain bulletproof throughout life, we need to keep a pep in our step and ensure we can absorb, transfer, and produce force without injuring ourselves. To be certain, crawling and walking do strengthen and nurture our slings, but they are "gentle" and are slower, low-force movements. We also want to be able to produce quick, powerful movements and we want our body to be used to doing this, so we don't ever ask it to do something it is not ready for.

Above, the only real place we have addressed the springiness of our springs is in the 10-minute jump rope from our *Tasks at Hand* section. This does address the springs and gets our muscles and tendons used to hopping and bouncing, but it doesn't really do much for the slings. If we want to address both at the same time, we need to look at marching, skipping, and bounding. All of these movements can be done "gently" and frequently in order to prepare the body to produce and absorb force.

These movements are in our gait pattern and each builds on the other. In truth, these movements are "crawling" on two feet, only quicker and "snappier". This is a bonus to us because not only do they strengthen our bodies on the outside, they also strengthen our nervous system on the inside, taking us closer and closer to becoming bulletproof. Adding a 10-minute session of these movements at the end of a training session twice a week can really add the finishing touch to our training as well as they can be quite the elixir — they make you feel good.

Here are a few sample Springs and Slings strength10me sessions you can add at the end of any training session:

Marching x <u>10 minutes</u> (this can be brutal in the beginning)

- Spread your fingers and sling your arms from your shoulders to match the swing of your hips.

- Make sure you land on the balls of your feet. Do not march on or from your heels.

- Keep your lips shut, your tongue on the roof of your mouth and breathe from your nose.

- Step quickly and with intent as if the ground is hot.

- Practice producing force once in a while — stomp the ground.

- Try to work up to ten continuous minutes using the same protocol for crawling.

A-Skipping x 10 minutes (also brutal in the beginning)

- A-skipping is marching with a small hop.

- Spread your fingers and sling your arms from your shoulders to match the swing of your hips.
  – Your movements should be crisp and quick.

- Hop about 1 to 2 inches from the ground with each step.

- Make sure you land on the balls of your feet. Do not skip on or from our heels.

- Keep your lips shut, your tongue on the roof of your mouth and breathe from your nose.

Skipping Session x 10 minutes

This is not a continuous skipping session, it is simply a timed event to work the springs and slings.

- Skip about 30 yards then walk back.

- Repeat this until 10 minutes expires.

- These are not necessarily A-skips, but regular skips you would make if you wanted to simply skip.

- USE your shoulders to match the movement and rhythm of your hips.

- Spread your fingers when skipping,

- Practice soft landings on the balls of your feet.

Bounding Session x 10 minutes

This is much like skipping, but different in that it is more purposeful and explosive. It may help to imagine leaping or bounding from rock to rock to cross a stream. It also may help to actually place targets or "lily pads" on the ground to get the feel of this as well as make it very fun and enjoyable.

- Bound about 30 yards then walk back.

- Repeat this until 10 minutes expires.

- USE your shoulders to match the movement and rhythm of your hips.
  – Drive those arms! They propel you and SLING you.

- Spread your fingers when bounding and leaping.

- Practice soft landings on the balls of your feet.

The Loose Structure of Seasons

Looking at the Becoming Bulletproof Training Template I presented above, you may be wondering, "Where is the structure?", "What day is chest day?", "When do we work the back?", or anything along those lines.

Don't think "exercise". If you only think in terms of "exercise" or if you only think from what you know about exercise, you'll miss the simple freedom and power in training like this. It is best to think through the lens of movement along with thinking in terms of work; showing up to do work and get stuff done. All the natural movements of the body are covered in the movement sessions above and you're not limited to the movements and tasks I've listed above. These are just big-bang-for-your-buck tasks and movements that will put you well on your way to becoming bulletproof. They work the mind and the body. You can certainly come up with different ones. Though I do encourage you to test yourself with the 10-minute tasks I've listed as being foundational.

Exercise thinking aside, there really is structure to the Becoming Bulletproof Template. It looks like this: Show up. Put in the time. Be consistent in showing up. Put in more time. All the while, practice managing your breathing by keeping your tongue on the roof of your mouth and filling your lungs up from the bottom to the top with your diaphragm.

That's it.

That's it?
This is really all you got?

This is how you develop work capacity and build both enduring strength and absolute strength. This is how hard things become easy and how uncomfortable things become comfortable — through showing up.

Having said that, you still need to use your brain, that muscle inside your head. There may be days you just need to show up and that is good enough. There may be days when you need to change the plan. There are no prizes to be won for working through pain and there are no trophies for not deviating from a plan. Use your intuition. If your mind or body is telling you something is "off" or "not right," it is okay to listen. I'm not talking about bowing down to weakness or laziness, I'm talking about not violating your internal alert system. Part of becoming bulletproof is knowing when to bend so that you don't break. Remember the rule of "doing what you can." There are simply going to be some days where you can do a great deal and then there are going to be other days when just showing up is good enough. There may even be days where you say, "Not today." I know, the horror...

Remember, training is not your identity. It is not who you are. At best it simply helps you learn, reveal or discover who you are. But it isn't you. It's just something you do to grow. It should enhance your life and make it better, it should never be your life. I've made that mistake. You don't need to. Got it?

Keep in mind too, that everything has a season. This is a wonderful lesson John Brookfield taught me. Nothing is meant to stay the same. Everything has a season and every season has a purpose: growth and becoming...

In the beginning of your bulletproof journey, there is a season of mental and physical struggle which is truly a season of growth. After a while though, as you get stronger the struggle goes away. Things do become easier if not just easy. You may then enter a season of "make it harder." You'll try to find clever ways of making things more difficult, so you can become even more bulletproof. This season is quickly followed by the season of burnout. You have made things so unpleasant, you lose your drive to engage and you start pondering other avenues. This is actually a good season because it brings you to the point of wondering, "How much is enough?" This is a great question to wrestle with.

So, how much is enough? When can you stop making things harder? When are you truly bulletproof? I'll talk more about this in the following chapters, but I'll give you some quick answers here.

To the age-old *often never pondered* question, "How much is enough?", I think the answer is when you no longer have anything left to prove to yourself. When you can let go of the false notion of perpetually making progress and discover that you are strong enough to live your life the way you want to. How much is enough gets answered when you can let go of the "strength opinions" of others and when you realize the only person qualified to answer this question is you. It happens when you discover there really is a margin of diminishing returns to everything, and you just need to be strong enough to live life on your terms. This is a season of huge reflection and growth.

This season leads to a knowing; a knowing that you are bulletproof, and you can do all things. You become bulletproof the moment you believe and know that you are bulletproof. What you hold in mind, you become. It's as simple as that. But let's talk about it.

I CAN

"*Indeed, there are two kinds of strength. The outer strength is obvious. It fades with age and succumbs to sickness. Then there is the Chi, the inner strength. Everyone possesses it, too, but it is much more difficult to develop. The inner strength lasts through every heat and every cold... Through old age and beyond.*"
— Master Kan, *Kung Fu*

To be sure, the Becoming Bulletproof Template in the previous chapter does develop both types of strength; mental and physical, or inner and outer. In looking at the quote above, yes, with time physical strength can lessen or fade. But mental strength or inner strength can undergird it through time and help preserve it beyond what is normal. And that is the secret to becoming bulletproof — the inner strength, your mind.

What your mind believes becomes. If you believe you are strong, you are strong. If you believe you are weak, you are weak. A fearful, stressed, apathetic, depressed mind leads to a dull, dark and dreary life. A bold, joyful, passionate mind leads to a vibrant, bright, adventurous life. The body follows the mind, as does the world around the mind.

Your mind, your thoughts and beliefs are more than powerful. They create how you perceive and experience the world around you and the life you live. Therefore, learning how to control your thoughts, learning how to set your mental GPS on a target and learning that you are capable of all things, is as essential to a healthy life as a healthy vestibular system is.

You must have inner strength to become bulletproof. You were made to have it, but you aren't required to have it. Just as you were made to be physically strong, but you're not required to be physically strong. Choice, discipline, training and intention all shape, guide and refine our inner strength, thus ultimately our physical strength.

There are other routes to developing your mental tenacity beyond the physical training mentioned above. Simply exposing yourself to unpleasant things can help build a type of "mental callus" that later protects your mind from would-be stressors while it bolsters your belief in your capacity to overcome anything. Regardless of the route you take to building your inner strength, that route must still be paved with intention, choice and discipline. "I can." And "I am" must be etched into your heart of hearts.

The Cold Buried Treasure

The truth is "I can" and "I am" are actually already etched into your heart. We talked about the hero in you gnawing to be revealed in the opening chapter of this book. Your inner superhero is screaming "I can!", "I'm here!", "I am able!" Chances are, if you're reading this book, you already know this. But what if the scream is faint and not heard? What if it's there but buried so deep you're just unaware? This is where introducing yourself to unpleasant things can help you find this treasure buried within. Let me explain.

Chances are you've heard of cold-water dousing, if not you may know it as The Ice Bucket Challenge. This became pretty popular about 5 years ago as a way to raise awareness and funds to support those with ALS. If you're unfamiliar, you take a 5-gallon bucket (or larger container), fill it with ice and water, and then dump it over your head. It's quite the refreshing treat — if you've ever wondered if you are alive, I encourage you to try this just once. You'll have no doubt that you are alive, if it doesn't kill you...

Anyway, about 2 to 3 years before the Ice Bucket Challenge was popular, John Brookfield encouraged me to engage in it because he believed it was a way to help one build mental toughness. Cold water dousing has other benefits as well, physical benefits, but the mental strength benefit is the apex. Just the shear will it takes to tip the bucket far enough over to spill its contents over your head almost seems to take an act of God. Oh man... But John had done this off and on over the years to harden his mind and he thought I should do it too as he was taking me under his wing.

So, one day when I was home alone — that was very important, my wife would not have understood — I filled up a bucket with ice and water, stepped into my shower, and tried to pour a bucket of water over my head. It seemed like it took me 20 minutes to get up the nerve, and that's all I felt when I finally tipped the bucket over my head: nerves. Every last nerve in my body was set on fire. Talk about an exhilarating rush! It was PHENOMENAL. I was alive. In fact, about 30 seconds after I poured the ice water over my head, something happened in my mind. I knew right then, I could do anything. It wasn't the "yeah, yeah, I can do anything I set my mind to do" knowing it was a deeper knowing of "Bring it. I can do it." That ice-cold bucket of water uncovered something in me — *knowing*...

That one event in my shower lead to a whole other type of training. It flipped a switch in me. From that day on, every day for a year, 365 days or more, I dumped a bucket of ice water over my head. No excuses, no exceptions. I did it at the fire station if I was at work. We had ice machines that made the small cubes. That was really nice! I did it in hotel room bathrooms if I was traveling; drove my wife crazy. All hotels had trashcans and ice machines. I always found a way because I was intent on finding a way. And at home, I would even do it outside in the dark on 15° mornings — before the neighbors were awake. It's funny how ice water feels warm when it's well below freezing outside. Anyway, every single day, I doused. And it was nothing. That exhilaration of that very first time was long gone, and cold-water dousing was just something I called "Tuesday". I tamed it. It didn't set my nerves on fire. My body didn't care, nor did my mind.

A year later, I stood with a bucket and thought, "Tim, you've nothing left to prove." So, I stopped. That was years ago. I know right now, if I wanted to, I could jump right back in and do it. YES, the first one would light me up like a Christmas tree, but only my body. My mind can do it, because I just said I could.

And that's the point. You can if you believe you can. You really can do anything. If you don't believe that, I encourage you to pour a bucket filled with ice and water over your head. As crazy as it sounds, it may uncover your inner knowing that *you can*. If you're really up to the challenge, I encourage you to try this every day for a month. You will learn so much about yourself, it's like discovering a treasure hidden in your own body.

Belief is Contagious

If the body follows what the mind believes, what happens when you don't believe anything, or you don't know what to believe? What I mean to say is that sometimes we simply don't know what we are capable of, so we don't necessarily believe anything positive about what we could do because we just don't know or because we lack creativity. Sometimes we need to borrow the belief of another.

I mentioned above that the world around you will also follow your beliefs. That means, the belief of others can and will shape your path as well. This is why it is so important to surround yourself with the type of people you want to be like. If you want to be strong — in every sense of the word — seek out strong people and hang around them. Let their beliefs influence your direction and your outcomes.

In a very simplistic example of this, the only reason I ever spider-man crawled for a mile is because John Brookfield casually told me one day, "You know Tim, I'll bet you could crawl a mile. You could do that." Before he said that, that had never been a thought in my head. I wasn't believing I could do it because I never imagined doing it. But as soon as John planted the seed that I could, through his belief in me, I began believing I could. And then I did — with NO specific training for it, other than holding the belief that I could do it. You see, John believed in me and I believed John. His belief bolstered mine. And I proved him right. I'll never forget what he said the day I told him I did it, I crawled a mile: "You know Tim, you should really have that on video. You should do it again and record it."

Ha! Wait, what?

John is sneaky. He gently encourages me, knowing my own ability better than I do, to push me further and further. And I end up wanting to, simply because he believes in me. I know I can, because he says I can and in some weird way, I don't want to let him down. So I end up doing something silly, like spider-man crawling a mile, twice…

Does this make sense? You're not meant to be isolated from the world. What good would it be to be the strongest person ever, or to be the ultimate superhero, with no one to share your gifts and experiences with? Who needs to be bulletproof if they stay away from people? Our true and full potential is born only to share it with others, only to help others. We actually give others our powers, especially our powers of belief. We can do more with others and because of others than we could ever do on our own. And it is often the compassion and belief of another that becomes the catalyst for us to discover our own potential.

I'll say it again, the beliefs we hold inside shape the world around us; they affect others. The belief of others also affects us. This is true in both a positive, potential discovering direction and also in a negative, potential oppressing direction. It is super important you hang out with the people who are shining the same light you want to become. The light and strength of others helps bulletproof and strengthen you. Conversely, the darkness and weakness of others can also be like kryptonite. Stay away from kryptonite.

Just on the chance that you have no one to lift you up, or on the chance that you are surrounded with negative thinking and negative believing people, I am telling you right now that you can become bulletproof. You can become a success. You can do anything — you do have the potential. I believe you can, and I know you can. You can…

Trusting in Something Bigger than Belief

All beliefs influence outcome. Even misplaced beliefs. Heck, it's why there is a placebo effect. A body can heal from a sugar pill if the person believes the sugar pill is the cure they need. Because of this, I *believe* it is of the utmost importance to saturate yourself with the right beliefs. Belief can take you a long way towards where you want to go, if used appropriately, especially when combined with knowing.

Sometimes belief needs help in the form of depth. Belief does have a depth to it. We can have shallow beliefs that can be easily unearthed and blown away or we can have deep rooted beliefs that can withstand an atomic bomb. How do we give depth to our beliefs? Through experience and knowing. Experience can actually bolster belief and bring you to knowledge; you can know things through experience. But there is another kind of knowing, a knowing where you just *know* that you know. This type of knowing is hard to achieve through rational thought, you don't necessarily find it or learn your way to it. It finds you. This knowing that finds you is like belief but at the same time it's not. It comes from within you, like a rising wellspring. It may seem like intuition or an unquestionable gut feeling or something deeper still. It comes to you through you. This knowing comes from a Source bigger than yourself — It's not you. Combined with belief, this knowing is immeasurably powerful.

Here's my story...

A few months after I asked God to show me how to train to become bulletproof, after I learned the miracles of crawling and revisiting the movements of a child, I was "frightened awake" by a dream I had around 3:00 am. I heard both a booming voice and saw a sign in my dream that said, "Wait on the Lord." It was loud. It scared me to the point that I jumped awake. Realizing it was a dream, I closed my eyes and immediately went back to sleep. Then BOOM, I had the same "dream" and heard the same voice, "Wait on the Lord." I looked around, saw my wife sleeping, thought I was weird, and went back to sleep. Then a third time, seconds later, "WAIT ON THE LORD!" I jumped up and said, "Ok!" I got out of bed, googled the phrase, "Wait on the Lord" and found Isaiah 40:31. Here's what it says:

"Those who wait on the Lord shall renew their strength. They shall rise up on wings like eagles. They shall run and not be weary. They shall walk and not faint."

I didn't know the depth of this verse that night/morning and I am still learning now, all these years later, its depth has no bottom. I will tell you though, this verse essentially says, "Those who wait on the Lord (those who look to God, who are aware of God, who TRUST God) shall become bulletproof." That's what it says, and that's what it means.

Ok, I am aware that some of you reading this may have different beliefs than I do. That is okay. I only ask that you not let the words "God" and "Lord" stop you from hearing what I'm saying. No one, myself included, can contain God in a name or a label. We can only use them to designate a path for our thoughts and intentions. Whether you prefer to use the words "God," "Universe," "Spirit," "Om," "Christ," "Holy One," "Creator" or whatever, I ask that you be open to the idea that you are not alone. You did not just *happen*. You are wonderfully designed by something Greater, and your Designer cares for you. Ok?

Whether you believe this to be true or not, I encourage you to meditate or marinate on these words: "Those who learn to trust in the Lord shall become bulletproof." Let them roll over and over in your head. Let them sink down into your heart. If you do, you may find that they rise up from your center as a knowing.

There are other verses in the Bible, and other places, that are just as powerful and beneficial to marinate over. I'll share some with you here.

- Philippians 4:13 — "I can do all things through Him who strengthens me."

- Joshua 1:9 — "This is my command--be strong and courageous! Do not be afraid or discouraged. For the LORD your God is with you wherever you go."

- Psalm 18:1 — "I love you, Lord; You are my strength."

- Isaiah 41:10 — "Don't be afraid, for I am with you. Don't be discouraged, for I am your God. I will strengthen you and help you. I will hold you up with my victorious right hand."

These verses, if you marinate on them, if they take root in you, they strengthen you. They produce a knowing in you. What if you knew that you were never alone? What if you knew that God, or the Creator of ALL there is, loved you and wanted to give you His strength? What if you knew, if you relied on His strength, and not your own, you really could do anything? What if...?

Ok, here is the rest of this story. Since that time, since that dream of Isaiah 40:31, I have experienced and discovered quite a few things. For one thing, I learned that Isaiah 40:28 says, "Have you never heard? Have you never understood? The LORD is the everlasting God, the Creator of all the earth. He never grows weak or weary." Compare that to Isaiah 40:31. Do you see it? Isaiah 40:31 not only says God will make you bulletproof, it says He'll make you like Him. Wow. Ok, sorry, that just fills me with hope.

I also learned or started believing I could cut out the "middle-man" in my pursuit to become bulletproof. If I relied on God to make me bulletproof, it took the pressure off me. Through some unusual circumstances here are some of the discoveries I made along the way. One day on a whim, I decided to attempt a 135-pound Turkish Get-up with a barbell. If you don't know what a Turkish Get-up is, it is holding a weight in an outstretched arm while lying on your back, then standing up with that weight while keeping it in your outstretched arm so that the weight is now overhead. Anyway, weighing 160 pounds myself, I decided to attempt this movement with 135 pounds on a barbell. That was 84% of my bodyweight held in one arm while I transitioned my body from lying to standing. If you've never done a getup with a barbell, that's a whole other animal than using a kettlebell or dumbbell... Oh, here's the real point of the story: I didn't practice get-ups — I hadn't done them in over a year.

Typically, when strength training, you practice the lifts you want to get stronger in. I hadn't practiced get-ups. In fact, and this is the "craziest" part, I had been using walking as my strength training regimen. I hadn't even been crawling for over a year. Truth — I took a year off from crawling. There is no reason I should have been able to perform this get-up. Yet, I did it. Twice. Once in each arm. I can only attribute this to the "whim," the knowing that came up inside me, and the Strength that could not have come from myself.

You see, I had started believing and knowing (that's the important part, the *and knowing* part) that my strength and ability didn't really come from what I was doing as much as they came from what (Who) I was believing.

The second time I crawled a mile, I also had the same knowing inside. Yes, John Brookfield believed I could do it, but to be honest, I didn't want to. I had already done it and while it was a "neat" thing to have accomplished, I can't say it really felt all that pleasurable. It certainly didn't feel pleasurable enough for me to ever want to do it again. So I sat alone the night

John told me to do it again and I just sat there thinking and meditating to God about it. And inside me, I had a knowing that He would hold me up in his right hand. And I also knew that I would do it much faster. I didn't know I would do it over 5 minutes faster than I did the first time. And the second time, it really wasn't all that uncomfortable at all. It was basically a crawl in the park...

Don't misunderstand me. I'm not suggesting you do nothing physical and simply believe you can do anything — though, you'll certainly be more capable with that belief. I did put in the work. I had spent a few years returning my Original Strength and while doing that I had engaged in the style of *becoming bulletproof* trainings I've illustrated above. I did build up a foundation — but that was training I was led to do anyway. So yes, I had learned how to condition my body and my mind with the uncomfortable. But while I was working on building the resiliency of my body and mind with this type of training, God was also working on building the strength of my inner self with His truths, strengthening my mind through belief and knowing, making me more resilient. Along the way, this gave me even more freedom and courage to explore and discover what I was capable of.

For example, I took over a year off of Battling Ropes — picked it up one day and performed 10 straight minutes of waves at 90 waves per minute. When I decided to crawl again, I easily crawled for 10 straight minutes — as if I never missed a day. I picked up a jump rope after years of not touching one and performed 10 straight minutes at 140 jumps per minute. I promise I'm not trying to boast, I'm only trying to illustrate how my ability remained — less from physical preparation and more from simply knowing and trusting, "I can."

And that's what I'm trying to get you to. If you get to the point where you just know, "I can," you're bulletproof. Nothing can phase you, nothing can stop you. You can do all things because not only have you prepared yourself to do them, you're trusting in a deeper Strength; a Strength you don't control but

[handwritten margin note: why were you taking so much time off from your system?]

allow to move through and from you. When you know you're not alone, when you learn how to trust in Strength beyond yourself, you are free to be bold and express yourself in every way you can imagine. Remember, those who learn to trust in the Lord shall become bulletproof...

Moving Meditation

There is another huge benefit in training to become bulletproof, especially if you train in blocks of time or you train to get tasks done. The becoming bulletproof sessions lend themselves well to meditation; a moving meditation.

Typically, meditation and soul reflection is done in solitude, stillness and quiet. It is a way, but not the only way. If you allow yourself the opportunity, you can perform all the tasks and training sessions alone, in quiet, and stillness of mind. If you do meditate, I'm not suggesting you replace your meditation with movement training. What I am suggesting is that if you don't meditate (and even if you do) you explore training and moving in silence, focusing on your breath, or the movements of your body, or even your thoughts. You can even focus on a verse, like the ones I listed above, while you move; running the verse over and over in your head while you get your work done.

Training this way and performing uncomfortable tasks in silence can become quite therapeutic. I am certain doing this has deepened my relationship with God. At moments when I was feeling the struggles of my body or mind, I would often begin to think on Him and His strength. It would carry me through. At other times, I would discover creative solutions or ideas for issues I was trying to solve, much like the epiphanies people report having while taking a shower. The point is, I would often leave training sessions feeling more deeply connected, rooted and grounded spiritually. And again, this left me with a knowing that "I can."

Training in silence also requires you to be internally driven. It makes you search your soul for drive. Music can be used to externally motivate people to move and do things. Podcasts ı distract from the physical discomfort. Listening to the news while you train will only feed your soul negativity, never do that! But silence, silence is the birth place of growth and discovery. It can help you find a Deeper part of yourself or a Bigger part of yourself that you were not aware of. It can help you discover that even though you are in the solitude of your mind, you are never truly alone. Nothing makes you more bulletproof than knowing this.

I know this is weird but give this a try. Remove all external distractions. Just you, your task and your silence. You will become even stronger if you learn to embrace this silence. It really can deepen your knowing of who you are and what you can do. It's like putting on an extra layer of Kevlar, making you even more bulletproof.

You are going to train in silence, maybe not all the time, but you are going to make this a part of your practice. Because you are serious about trying this, you are going to put earplugs in your ears — just do it, it's crazy enough to work.

How do I know you will do this? Well, if you're reading this book, you want to become bulletproof. That also means you are intent on becoming bulletproof. Which means you will become bulletproof. Which means you will be training in silence...

no I'm NOT.."

BULLETPROOF NUTRITION

"It's not what goes into your mouth that defiles you; you are defiled by the words that come out of your mouth."
— Matthew 15:11 NLT

"...What you say flows from what is in your heart."
— Luke 6:45 NLT

You can strengthen your mind and your body through what you think, how you think, how you move and through what you believe. But is there a way to eat, a lifestyle eating plan, that will help you on your journey to becoming bulletproof?

Yes, I think there is, and I'll share it with you here. However, it stems more from what you believe than it does from what you eat. In the previous chapter, we discussed the power of belief. Belief can AND will play a huge role in your nutritional well-being. Notice I used the words "nutritional well-being." The health of nutrition doesn't just come from food, it also comes from your thoughts about food. What you believe about food will affect your mental and physical well-being. It will either set you free or imprison you. If you are free, you are bulletproof. If you are imprisoned, you are vulnerable. Let's take a look...

The body needs food. Food fuels and nourishes us. It keeps us alive and helps our bodies carry out their functions like thought, cell division, cell repair, respiration, digestion (duh), movement and whatever else the body does. ALL food can play a part in this, even "bad" food.

So, let's start here. "Bad" food is a label. We label food as good or bad, healthy or not healthy, wholesome or even evil. We label the food and we then act on the belief in the label. But food really isn't good or bad in as much as food just is. I understand that some will point to poisonous foods as being bad, but I would counter that if it is poisonous food, it is not food. Anyway, what we label as bad or good is very subjective and likely to be situationally true.

For example, most people probably wouldn't have a problem saying that sugar is bad for you. Those people would probably classify a lollipop as a "bad" food. But for a person about to go into a hypoglycemic coma (diabetic coma) a lollipop could save their life — not in a permanent solution sense but a temporary intervention sense. The point is that at the appropriate time, in a given situation, a "bad" food could suddenly become "good." And the bigger point is food is more than the labels we put on it. But we tend to operate from the labels we place on food because the labels influence our beliefs and our beliefs influence our outcomes.

So, a place to start when pondering if food can help us become bulletproof, is probably to drop the labels or at the very least look at food along a spectrum or sliding scale: Good, better, best. And it is a sliding scale based on what is optimal from what is available in the moment of need. What is the need? To eat.

Ok, labels are out (maybe), but what about diets, or "ways" of eating? What about fasting and macronutrient ratios? What about eating like cavemen or less than modern Mediterranean civilizations? What about grains, fruit, or paleo cookies? What about all the rules? Don't eat after midnight, don't get them wet. Oh, sorry. We aren't gremlins. But what about Ketosis, carb loading, protein depletion, catabolism and anabolism? What about phytoestrogens, GMO's, organics, free-range, true free-range, pasture raised, Omega-6s, molds, phytochemicals, xenoestrogens, transfats, extra-virgin cold pressed, heat processed, chemical extraction, and food allergies.

These are all things to consider — or not. The answer to any of these and all of these lives more in what you believe about them than anything else. Your belief system about food constructs the framework from which you will operate and this will produce the outcome you experience — the outcome you want or the outcome you don't want.

I'm not saying the questions and issues above aren't real or valid, I'm saying the beliefs behind them yield the experience. For example, take any diet and all its rules. Do the rules set you free or do they imprison you and make you miserable. Are you free to eat with friends you haven't seen in years or do you need to wait until the appropriate feeding time? Do you even respect the rules or intent of the diet or do you look for creative ways to make cookies out of bark, root and nut powder? Do you see what I mean about the beliefs and the framework they create? Our beliefs over food will cause us to go through enormous suffering and go through enormous lengths to play the game of the diet. It's all a trap.

Then there is the whole physical health cascade these nutrition beliefs affect. How much nutrition could you get out of the most nutrient dense food in the world if you were releasing a flood of adrenaline while eating this food BELIEVING you should not be eating until after your 16 hour fast window was to take place? Wait, what? Here's the deal, most people's beliefs over food cause them to stress over food. Stress over food influences the autonomic nervous system and can put a person in fight or flight mode instead of rest and digest mode. If you can't digest your food well because you're too busy fighting your thoughts about it, you're not going to get all you need from it — nutrient wise or soul wise.

To look at the other extreme, do you think a person could digest a cookie efficiently and maybe put that energy to good use if he were to eat it without a care in the world, simply enjoying the cookie? No stress. Just joy and freedom...

I'm not suggesting you eat cookies. I'm suggesting you examine your beliefs about food and come to a place where YOU have peace about the food you decide to eat or when you decide to eat it. You can be aware of all the rules and labels and toxins and ratios, but in the end, you simply have to be at peace with your choices KNOWING you are choosing to do the best you can with the resources you have. Is organic better than conventional? Not if you can't find it or buy it. Is grass-fed better than grain-fed? Does the answer mean you'll skip a soul and body nourishing meal if you are determined grain-fed beef is toxic?

I know, that sounds extreme. But when it comes to food and eating — people tend to swing to the extremes instead of finding life in the middle.

Take everything I've said, or not said really, with a grain of salt and don't forget that you were blessed with a mind, a tool for you to use, when it comes to determining the best path for you to travel. Use your brain and rationally determine the best way for you to eat. And don't lie to yourself — honestly approach your nutrition.

Here are some helpful ponderings and tips to get your mind working:

- Is the food in its natural state or did man put a great deal of chemicals in it or did man use a great deal of processing to present it? In other words, did God create it or is it an edible invention?

- Is the food in a cardboard box?

- Could it have ever been found in nature?

- Does the food expire quickly and naturally? It's probably nutritious if it does.

- Will the food last for years? Is it preserved? Do you need to eat embalmed food?

- Is it vibrantly colorful — on its own? Is it colored with man made concoctions?

- Carbs, Protein and Fat — eat those.

- Drink water

- How do you feel after you eat the foods you chose to eat? Do you feel good? Do you feel blah? If it makes you feel blah, should you eat it?

- Do you eat when you get hungry? Do you eat because you are hungry?

- Are you hungry? Should you just eat?

- Does food rule your thoughts? Does it consume your mental energy throughout the day? Do you think it should?

- Shop the edges of most stores and stay out of the aisles of most stores.

- Food is seasonal. In nature, food arrives in seasons and set periods. In stores, there is no season. Hmmmm....

- You too may have seasons of eating. There may be periods when a certain way or style of eating is really beneficial for you. That beneficial season may serve its purpose and pass, making room for a new season.

- Try new foods. Be curious about food and don't prejudge or label it with absolutely no personal experience.

- Taste buds are gifts. Appreciate them and allow them to help you discover the art of eating flavorful food.

- Wash your produce.

- Wash your hands.

- No matter what you say, the first meal of your day is technically breakfast (breaking the fast).

- Different regions and different genetics allow for different styles of eating that work really well for those specific groups or individuals. There is no blanket meal plan that fits everyone.

- The clock is just a clock. Use it to tell time and don't let it become the walls or laws you live to eat by.

- Should we go through life counting calories and eating to certain ratios of macronutrients? Is it really supposed to be this complicated?

- Shouldn't we enjoy eating? Shouldn't we enjoy eating with others?

- Instead of living to eat, or trying to eat to live, why not live to learn and then learn to eat?

- Be thankful for the food you eat.

This isn't an exhaustive list of ponderings and tips but it should get your wheels turning. In the end, you've got to find what works for you and you've got to come to a point where you are mentally free or judgement free of your food decisions and actions. If eating the "wrong" food at the "wrong" time causes you mental stress and turmoil, you may need to examine your food beliefs or their underlying fears. Eating should not be a stressor. It should be enjoyed.

Our thoughts truly influence our outcomes, in everything, even in how we digest and use the fuels we consume. So because of that, because the body follows the mind and what comes out of a person's heart is what defiles the person, what would happen if we ate with the belief we were gifting our body food? What if we ate believing we were doing something good for our body? What if we ate believing this food was going to help us achieve our strength, health and life goals? What would happen if we approached food that way. What if saying the blessing was less of a ritual and more of a declaration? I know it is crazy, but it just might be crazy enough to work...

BECOMING BULLETPROOF WITH "TRADITIONAL" TRAINING

"You got your peanut butter on my chocolate!" and the other would exclaim, "You got your chocolate in my peanut butter!"
— Reese's Peanut Butter Cup commercials, circa 1980s

You may be a person who enjoys traditional strength training but you also want to realize and release your inner super hero. You might be wondering if you can combine traditional strength training with the bulletproof type training I've outlined above. I've got good news for you friend; Yes, yes you can.

I understand that "traditional" strength training may have different definitions or opinions as to what it is, but that is okay. Just use your definition here. You can really do quite well combining traditional strength training with two to three days of becoming bulletproof training. In fact, you may get to the point where you think your traditional training days are "easy" days because they seem so laid back. Even if that's not the case, an every-other-day approach to combining traditional strength training and becoming bulletproof training is very doable and can yield some fantastic results. You may find your strength and performance reach never before achieved levels, especially if you are doing a great deal of crawling and loaded walking in your bulletproof training. This is because when you load the gait pattern, you tie the body together and take the brakes off the nervous system. In doing so, your strength and movement quality in the gym improves by leaps and bounds — you're becoming bulletproof...

How you combine your training is really up to your individual needs and schedule. I'll just provide some simple options here:

Traditional Bulletproofing

<u>Example 1</u>

Mondays — Chest day (couldn't resist) and all the compliments

- Press RESET x 10 minutes
- Your routine
- Press RESET x 5 minutes

Tuesdays

- Press RESET x 10 minutes
- Leopard Crawl x 10 minutes of work
- Chest Carries x 10 minutes
- Rucking x 20 to 30 minutes

Wednesday — Squat day

- Press RESET x 10 minutes
- Your routine
- Press RESET x 5 minutes

Thursday

- Press RESET x 10 minutes
- Backward Leopard Crawl x 10 minutes
- Sledge Hammer work x 10 minutes
- Sandbag Shoulder Carries x 10 minutes

Friday — Deadlift day

- Press RESET x 10 minutes
- Your routine
- Press RESET x 5 minutes

Example 2

Mondays — Deadlift and Back

- Press RESET x 10 minutes
- Your routine
- Press RESET x 5 minutes

Tuesday

- Press RESET x 10 minutes
- Weight of Water x 20 minutes
- Ruck Walk with loaded pack x 20 minutes

Wednesday

- Press RESET x 10 minutes
- Sled work x 15 minutes
- Chest Carries x 10 minutes
- Backward Leopard Crawl x 10 minutes

Thursday — Squat and Press

- Press RESET x 10 minutes
- Your routine
- Press RESET x 5 minutes

Friday

- Press RESET x 10 minutes
- Battling Ropes x 10 minutes
- Sandbag Getups x 10 minutes
- Suitcase Carries x 10 minutes
- Leopard Crawl x 10 minutes

Kettlebell Bulletproofing

<u>Example 1</u>

Monday

- Press RESET x 10 minutes
- Swings and Pullups x 10 minutes of escalating density training (getting as many sets of each done as you can in the time frame — <u>you</u> determine the reps in the set)
- Battling Ropes x 10 minutes of accumulated or continuous work depending on fitness level
- Leopard Crawl x 10 minutes of accumulated or continuous work

Tuesday

- Press RESET x 10 minutes
- Squats and Presses x 15 minutes of escalating density training
- Suitcase Carries x 10 minutes
- Ruck Walk x 20 minutes

Wednesday

- Press RESET x 10 minutes
- Turkish Getups x 10 minutes — your way
- Weight of Water x 10 minutes
- Kettlebell Rack Carries x 10 minutes

Thursday

- Press RESET x 10 minutes
- Snatches and Chin-ups x 10 minutes of escalating density training
- Battling Ropes x 10 minutes of accumulated or continuous work depending on fitness level
- Backward Leopard Crawl x 10 minutes of accumulated or continuous work

Friday

- Press RESET x 10 minutes
- Cleans to Squat to Press x 15 minutes of escalating density training
- Chest Carries x 10 minutes
- Ruck Walk with loaded pack x 20 minutes

<u>Example 2</u>

Monday — Bells

- Press RESET x 10 minutes
- Swings x 15 minutes of escalating density training in sets of 10
- Turkish Getups x 15 minutes of escalating density training (but do not rush) in sets of 3 per side
- Press RESET x 5 minutes

Tuesday — Bulletproofing

- Press RESET x 10 minutes
- Battling Ropes x 10 minutes of accumulated or continuous work depending on fitness level
- Leopard Crawl x 10 minutes of accumulated or continuous work
- Ruck Walk with loaded pack x 20 minutes

Wednesday — Bells

- Press RESET x 10 minutes
- Goblet Squats or Double Front Squats x 15 minutes, sets of 5 or 3
- Clean and Presses or Double Clean and Presses x 15 minutes, sets of 5 or 3
- Press RESET x 5 minutes

Thursday — Bulletproofing

- Press RESET x 10 minutes
- Suitcase Carries x 10 minutes
- Chest Carries x 10 minutes
- Sled work x 10 minutes
- Backward Leopard Crawl x 10 minutes

Friday — Bells

- Press RESET x 10 minutes

- Snatch, Squat, Long Push Press x 15 minutes, sets of 5 per side
  – Snatch a bell, pull it down to the rack position
  – Squat the bell
  – Stand up from the squat pushing the bell up overhead
  – You're very welcome

- Turkish Getups to the elbow position x 10 minutes, sets of 5 per side
  – Just sitting up to the elbow post position and then lying back to your back

- Press RESET x 5 minutes

Saturday — Bulletproofing Bonus

- Press RESET x 10 minutes
- Battling Ropes x 10 minutes of accumulated or continuous work depending on fitness level
- Sled work x 10 minutes

- SLOW MOTION Leopard Crawl x 15 minutes of accumulated or continuous work

Sunday — Bulletproofing Bonus

- Press RESET x 10 minutes
- Light Ruck with a loaded pack x 30 to 40 minutes

Please keep in mind that these are just options and examples. The combination of ways to pair bulletproof training with your desired way of training are too numerous to list here. Just keep in mind your goal; what you want out of your training, or more importantly, what you want out of your life. How do you want to feel? What do you want to do? Let those two questions help you carve out your training path here. When in doubt, load your gait pattern frequently (crawl, march, ruck, etc...). Just make it miserable!

Becoming Bulletproof on the Road

Some of us travel a lot. Traveling can put a kink into your training plans, but it doesn't have to. After all, if you are of the mindset you want to become bulletproof, traveling and living in hotels or guest rooms isn't even an obstacle, it's an opportunity.

With your intention and a little bit of space, you can still train to become bulletproof with absolutely zero training equipment. The following tasks make perfect close quarters (hotel room/bedroom), body-only training sessions. I'll present them in 10-minute sessions, though you could easily lengthen them. Picking and performing 2 to 5 of these tasks can make a great bulletproof training event that can easily be done every day you are away.

Body-only Bulletproofing — Pick two to five for a great movement session at home or on the road.

- Press Reset x 10 minutes
  - Begin each session with this.
  - Don't skip this.

- Be honest, this may be the only time you deliberately practice breathing with your diaphragm.

- Bodyweight Getups and Getdowns x 10 minutes
  - Lie on your back, roll to your belly and stand up.
  - Be creative.
  - Try to keep moving without resting.
  - You can also lie on your belly, roll to your back and stand up.
  - To challenge yourself, remove limbs (don't use your arms, your right leg, or whatever...)

- Leopard Crawl (or any crawl) x 10 minutes
  - If you've got the room, even if only for 5 steps, crawl forward and backward for time.
  - Can be practiced in slow motion or regular speed.
  - Keep those lips shut!!!

- Elevated Rock x 10 minutes (Brutal)
  - Get on your hands and knees with your feet dorsiflexed (ball of foot on floor). Then pick your knees just up off the floor.
  - Rock back and forth. For 10 minutes. Don't stop. Unless you have to.
  - You're welcome.

- Cross-crawls on your hands and feet x 10 minutes
  - If you have absolutely no room at all to crawl, but you have room to get on your hands and knees. You'll love this.
  - Get in the Leopard Crawl position and perform cross-crawl touches. These can be hand to thigh or elbow to knee.
  - In 10 minutes, you should be able to get about 330 touches at a comfortable pace.

- Standing Cross-Crawls x 10 minutes
  - I'm not even joking. I do this very often.
  - Try to touch your opposite arm to opposite leg for 10 minutes of continuous moving.
  - Hello core and hips!

- Squat and Pushup Mountain from 1 to 10 to 1
  - Same as described above only the squats are body-weight squats.
  - Can be any kind of pushup or squat (Hindu, tradition-al, split stance, etc...)
  - Get after it. Can you complete this in 15 minutes?

- Deadbugs x 10 minutes

- Elevated Speed-Skaters x 10 minutes
  - These are absolutely fantastic. Especially for those of you thinking, "But what about my back?" You will love what they do for you — after you're done with them.
  - Get on all fours as if you're going to Leopard Crawl.
  - Lift your opposite arm and leg together, both pointing back behind you.
  - Stay in one place. No need to move, though you can.

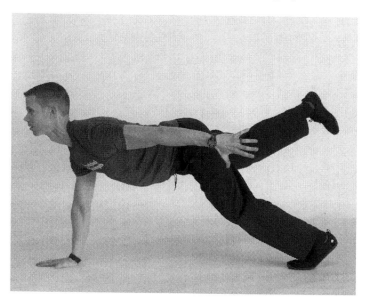

- Axis Crawls x 10 minutes
  - Get on all fours and imagine there is a pole going through your navel. Crawl in circles by spinning on your axis. Your navel should remain over the same

point on the floor while you spin, moving your opposite limbs together.

- Single Leg Deadlifts or Reverse Lunges x 10 minutes
  – Keep moving. Enjoy.

- Stairs and Hallways x 10 minutes
  – If you get up early enough, you can crawl, march, or skip down the hallways without anyone ever knowing. Even if they do know though, who cares?
  – You can always climb up and down the stairs practicing fast feet going up each stair or taking big steps covering 2 to 3 stairs at a time. On the way down, just be smart.

IT'S IN YOUR DESIGN

"It'd be a huge burden for anyone to bear; but you're not just anyone, Clark, and I have to believe that you were... that you were sent here for a reason. All these changes that you're going through, one day... one day you're gonna think of them as a blessing; and when that day comes, you're gonna have to make a choice... a choice of whether to stand proud in front of the human race or not." — Jonathon Kent, Man of Steel

As I said in the beginning of this book, The Becoming Bulletproof Project is about becoming who we were meant to be. More pointedly, it is about realizing who we actually are.

I believe the design of a thing determines the purpose of a thing. We create things for a certain function and purpose. We create cars for transportation, computers for computing and communication, homes for living in, and art for sharing beauty. Everything we design has a purpose, if for no other purpose than for experiencing the joy of creating something. We are no different.

Look at your design. Look at the wonder that encompasses you; how you move, how you think, how you can move, how you can think. Ponder the nerves that carry the information from your body to your brain and then the nerves that carry the commands from your brain to your body. Ponder where your thoughts come from; how you control them or how you don't control them. Ponder your emotions and those inner tugs and nudges you get; the ones you acknowledge and the ones you try to dismiss. Do you see the wonder? Do you see the potential? Your design screams that you are to have many purposes that all point to one singular purpose. You are clearly made to move, smile, think, create, love, play, work, heal, give and save. You are clearly made to share yourself with the world. This is how you save the day.

This is why it is so evident that you are meant to be bulletproof. You cannot share yourself, you can't give yourself, if you are afraid, weak, fragile or broken. You can't shine and smile and love if you are in the dark.

But, if you honor your design and all that was put in you; if you move well, think with strength, and realize and know that you are indeed someone who was designed to give themselves to the world — you are indeed a hero, you will begin to understand that you have no limitations and there is simply nothing you cannot do. You will know no obstacles but only opportunities. You will know that you were made to be strong, if for no other reason than the sheer joy your life creates in the world. That's who you are — the bulletproof hero, put here to save the world...

This book, the method, tasks and routines it contains are just to help you realize what you are capable of, to help you understand the potentiality of what you possess. If you know you can routinely make the hard things easy, the impossible things possible, you remove limitations. If you know you can overcome challenges and feel stronger with each challenge, you might begin to realize the truth: you are strong, but not because of the things you do but because of who you are.

You were created to be bulletproof. It's in your design. It's who you are, even if you don't realize it yet. Not knowing who you are doesn't change who you are. It just means you don't get to enjoy who you were meant to be. Anyway, it's up to you to engage in and embrace your design. It's up to you to answer that nudge inside of you, that gnawing to rise up and be more. The world is waiting for you to realize who you are. The world is waiting for its hero...

THE POTENTIAL OF
THE DESIGN

The following articles come from my website. I wrote them regarding some of my training experiences. I'm including them here as you may find them helpful in wrapping your head around what is possible in the journey to becoming bulletproof and realizing who you are.

How To Crawl a Mile

I crawled a mile once, ok maybe twice. I don't really talk much about it publicly, but once in a while, it comes up. My friend, Chad Faulkner, also crawled a mile and for whatever reason he and I were both talking about our mile experience last week and how we prepared to accomplish our task.

For me, personally, I never sat out to crawl a mile. It just kind of came up. I had been enjoying crawling for quite some time and for "fun" I had begun crawling 40 to 50 minutes at a time; not all the time, but once in a while. It was fun for me because I enjoyed the challenge and the looks of people's faces in the neighborhood. If you want to make yourself known, go crawl in public frequently. Everyone will know who you are, or they'll know about you at least. Anyway, I had become infatuated with crawling. I loved doing it and it seemed to love me back. It just made me feel amazing.

One day, while talking to another friend, John Brookfield, about my love for crawling, John said, "I'll bet you can crawl a mile. You should probably do that." That was it. The seed was planted. I hadn't thought about it until John mentioned it. But once John said it, I knew I could do it. Well, I believed I could if I relied on a strength beyond myself. And that's my secret. I believed. Was it difficult? A little. Was it uncomfortable? The first time it was. Did I train for it? That's debatable. I had gotten used to being uncomfortable by crawling for extended periods of time, but I never crawled close to a mile without stopping. And though all that time spent crawling did strengthen my body beyond my wildest expectations, it also strengthened my mind and my relationship.

Relationship? It's pretty difficult to crawl for time or distance without talking to yourself, or someone beyond yourself. To put it plainly, I had lots of conversations with God when I crawled. Some were with words and others were just a knowing that I wasn't alone; which is so wonderful to know. You can wonder if you're crazy or alone when you do weird things and it's nice to know you're not alone, just crazy! Anyway, through all my crawling and time spent crawling I began to believe I could do anything if God helped me to do it. That belief carried me a mile on my hands and feet, with my butt held down below my head, while I breathed through my nose. That belief carried me a mile, and beyond…

My friend, Chad, had a similar experience because he too had the same belief. He believed he could do it and he believed he would have help doing it. And he did.

By the way, crawling a mile (*Here is a video just in case you wanted to see it: https://www.youtube.com/watch?v=x0DtQ-YBnK4)* is just nuts. But so is running a marathon or competing in a triathlon. But I think sometimes we are called to be a little nuts because often we really don't know what we are capable of until something inside of us prods us along, until the relationship invites us to explore our own limits and move beyond them.

The point is, we can do anything we set out to do. If we rely on more than ourselves, and we believe. I really do believe all things are possible to him who believes — that he/she is not alone. The greatest limitations we have are the ones we place on ourselves through doubt and isolation. If we don't believe something is possible, we secure that impossibility by placing a limit on it. If we don't believe there is a Source greater than ourselves that wants to carry us along, we turn away from the help we need, and we cut ourselves off from limitless potential.

Here's the take home message on how to crawl a mile, or any other insane thing:

You were made to be limitless.

You can do anything you set your mind to do.

You're not alone.

Believe it.

Does Training Have to Hurt?

A good friend of mine and I decided to do an experiment. We wanted to see if it were possible to train for a half Ironman triathlon without hurting her body or her performance at work. In the past when she had trained for such races, her training was very demanding, and it took a toll on her body, her mind and her job. She was using so much energy to train and recover, she was having a hard time focusing on and giving herself to her clients at work. So, the question was, "Is it possible to train for a half Ironman without the training being so consuming, so she could physically feel good, mentally perform at work, and yet still be competitive and perform well in her race?" The answer was, "Yes. Yes, it is!"

If you don't know, a half Ironman consists of a 1.2-mile swim, a 56-mile bike ride and a 13.1-mile run. To be honest, I would not want to engage in any one of those tasks alone, let alone combine them all in one event. Triathletes are truly special and gifted people. Anyway, the physical stamina and mental tenacity it requires to complete such a task is tremendous. Typically, from what I understand the training frequency and volume to complete such races, half or full triathlons, is fairly demanding — especially if you have a full-time job and life outside of your training. Before I go further, I understand there are many different approaches and methods for approaching training for triathlons. But what we really wanted to know is could we wrap the majority of training inside of an Original Strength and Easy Strength method so that my friend could have easy to moderate training days and one really good race day. You know, one day to survive (race day), rather than hundreds of days to survive (training days).

So that was the experiment. We laced my friend's training with the Original Strength resets and an Easy Strength Mindset. Every day of the week she pressed reset in various forms, for time, like rolling for 10 minutes, crawling for 10 minutes, etc. Every other day we engaged in one of the events she would be performing in the race, but we did it with very low intensity, like running one to three miles, or just spending time in the water, "feeling" the water and dialing in her strokes, or getting on the bike with friends for weekend rides that lasted between one to two hours. On days we did not engage in swimming, biking and running, we did lots of loaded carries like walking with a backpack for time. In everything we did, we practiced nasal breathing with her lips closed, getting her diaphragm strong while making her lungs and heart efficient. Unless she was on a weekend ride with friends, training rarely lasted an hour.

The results? Well, her body never broke down. Her mind never tapped out. She felt good on most days and was able to completely give herself to her patients at work. She was also able to give herself to her friends and enjoy a social life. She wasn't consumed with training or recovering from training. Oh, and on race day? She did fantastic. She crushed her events and had one of the best experiences and "highs" of her life. And that makes me happy...

Again, I know there are several ways to skin a cat. But what if you could be as strong as you wanted to be, perform as well as you wanted to in your sport, and live the life you wanted to live through simply rubbing the cat instead of skinning it? What if training didn't have to hurt? What if training felt good and built you up? What if we changed the way we view training? What if instead of trying to build the body up by conventional means to add more strength, power and stamina, we simply cut the cords and removed the brakes that were holding the body back, allowing it to express untapped strength, power and stamina?

I'm not suggesting training will never be tough or should never be. I'm only pondering and experiencing that maybe a little training goes a lot further when the body has no limits placed on it. Maybe training is more effective, or a smaller dose is needed, when the body is moving and performing optimally. Maybe training isn't smothering we survive through in hopes of performing well but something we thrive through in confidence of optimally performing.

The point is training doesn't have to hurt. And, rubbing the cat may be a lot better than skinning it...

How I Trained for the RKC without Using Kettlebells

I recently attended an RKC kettlebell certification. It was a recertification for me. To be honest, the reason I really wanted to attend was because it was being taught by Master Instructor, Dan John. Dan is a wealth of coaching wisdom and I wanted to see what I could glean from him. Anyway, the RKC certification is a three-day kettlebell cert that includes various skill and technique tests with the kettlebell as well as the infamous 100 snatches in five minutes test and the "graduation" workout. These last two things alone, are enough to make you dig deep into your soul and ponder if you're making the right life decisions.

To survive such a weekend filled with some intense challenges is an accomplishment. The first time I "survived" the

RKC certification was in 2006. I remember it very vividly still today. I trained for several months to be able to endure the certification. Thankfully, my training paid off. I did indeed survive.

Coming into this cert was different though, and it had some new challenges of its own. One, I really *really* wanted to learn from Dan John, to understand how he thinks and teaches. Two, I don't want to survive my way through a cert. I want to thrive, and I want to learn. Surviving usually puts learning in the back seat. And three, I don't really train with kettlebells or weights anymore and I'm 11 years older than the first time I survived the RKC.

I know what you're thinking. Points two and three are greatly at odds with each other. How can I expect to thrive through an intense three-day kettlebell certification and not ready myself by planning/practicing/training with kettlebells? Well, it's simple. I have my Original Strength.

I currently have two driving principles in my life. These two principles help guide my training and movement choices.

1) It feels good to feel good. I believe this with all my heart. If I do something that doesn't feel good, or doesn't allow me to feel good, I probably don't need to do it. Conversely, if I find something that feels good and enables me to feel good and enjoy my life, I should probably hold on to it.

2) I want to make the hard things easy. If I can train in such a way that hard things become easy, then nothing is hard. And then, on that day when I really come across something that truly is hard, I should have extra reserves in my mind and body to step up to the task.

These two principles, along with the influence of my friends, Dan John and John Brookfield, also shape the way I train. Before I tell you how I train, I should tell you that I did indeed thrive through the RKC weekend. In fact, every morning before the day would begin, I would engage in my own "exercise" routine. I use that word loosely, but you would call it exercise or a workout. Yes, I worked out each day of the RKC before the day actually began...

Anyway, I enjoyed my RKC experience and I soared through its challenges, effortlessly. Without training with kettlebells, or weight lifting. Here is what I did.

EVERY DAY, because it is important to my number one guiding principle, I Press RESET. I breathe, I nod my head, I rock, I roll, and I crawl or march or walk. Every day. AND, every day, I perform some type of carry or loaded gait pattern. I may go for a 30-minute walk with my heavy backpack, or I may crawl backward while I pull a sled. But the point is, I load my gait pattern every single day, if only for a few minutes. Well, Sunday is an exception. Sunday's I typically just roll around on the floor for 10 minutes or take a walk. But every day, other than Sunday, I do these things. By the way, loading my gait pattern is where I learned to make the hard things easy. Carrying a heavy load for time and distance, or crawling across a football field dragging 100 pounds, hardens your mind and body. It quickly takes the breaks off your ability to perform difficult things — while it makes you ridiculously strong...

And to be completely transparent, I also currently perform 100 hindu pushups (they are a RESET) and 100 hindu squats every day.

And that, that is my secret sauce (along with another factor — my beliefs) for being able to thrive through the RKC certification without training with kettlebells. The RESETs allow me to move effortlessly and efficiently, giving me the ability to guide the kettlebell where it needed to be to perform the swings, snatches, cleans, getups and squats. The carries gave me the strength, stamina, and mental advantage to crush the reps, sets, tests and workouts — with my lips closed, breathing in and out through my nose.

That's Being Bulletproof

Being able to thrive through trials is the essence of being bulletproof. In the above article about attending the RKC certification, being bulletproof gave me the ability to focus on the instruction of Dan John *and* learn from the kettlebells themselves. I was able to focus and learn because I was never in any mental distress because my body wasn't trying to survive. I was attacking physical challenges with joy and learning inside the movements, constantly evaluating them and the sensations of my body. I was actually able to dance with the kettlebells and flow with them, making the movements look effortless. This is what movement and training is all about, being able to live life better because you can enjoy it, because you can move and think your way through it.

Please understand, my point is not to say you don't need to train with weights or kettlebells. My point is to say if you know you are bulletproof, you can train with anything you want, and you can enjoy it. Becoming bulletproof allows you to live your life better. It allows you to feel good, which feels good. It allows you to make the hard things easy and even enjoyable. It enables you to thrive through the trials that will test you without breaking your body or panicking your mind.

Again, that's the essence of becoming bulletproof and it keeps building on itself. Thriving through trials builds even more endurance, which develops your character even more, which builds a hope in you that knows no bounds.

Endurance, character and hope — The marks of a bulletproof hero...

REFERENCES

1. https://www.ncbi.nlm.nih.gov/pmc/articles/PMC3731110/

2. https://www.ncbi.nlm.nih.gov/pmc/articles/PMC3940506/

3. https://www.youtube.com/channel/
   UCC6g6yv0bSnA6nO3glRKL_Q

Learn More About Original Strength

Original Strength is an education company who teaches about the power of human movement. Our company's vision is to inspire every professional who places their trust in us to live boldly and utilize their professional Original Strength Certifications in their own business as Personal Trainers, Physical Therapists, Chiropractors, Wellness & Strength Coaches, K-12 Educators, and many other professions.

The Original Strength team invites you to visit our website at OriginalStrength.net for more information on these revolutionary human movement products: Videos, Books, DVDs, and Equipment.

To find a workshop near you please visit OriginalStrength.net/events.

To find an Original Strength Certified Professional near you visit: Originalstrength.net/find-a-certified-coach

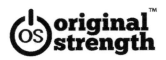

"...I am fearfully and wonderfully made..."
Psalm 139:14

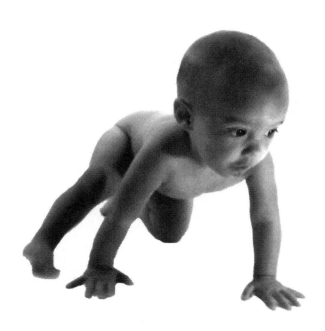

Made in the USA
Columbia, SC
22 May 2019